Painscapes

EJ Gonzalez-Polledo • Jen Tarr
Editors

Painscapes

Communicating Pain

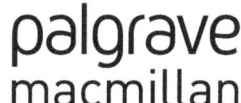

Editors
EJ Gonzalez-Polledo
Department of Anthropology
Goldsmiths, University of London
London, UK

Jen Tarr
London School of Economics and Political Science
London, UK

ISBN 978-1-349-95271-7   ISBN 978-1-349-95272-4 (eBook)
https://doi.org/10.1057/978-1-349-95272-4

Library of Congress Control Number: 2017950172

© The Editor(s) (if applicable) and The Author(s) 2018
The author(s) has/have asserted their right(s) to be identified as the author(s) of this work in accordance with the Copyright, Designs and Patents Act 1988.
This work is subject to copyright. All rights are solely and exclusively licensed by the Publisher, whether the whole or part of the material is concerned, specifically the rights of translation, reprinting, reuse of illustrations, recitation, broadcasting, reproduction on microfilms or in any other physical way, and transmission or information storage and retrieval, electronic adaptation, computer software, or by similar or dissimilar methodology now known or hereafter developed.
The use of general descriptive names, registered names, trademarks, service marks, etc. in this publication does not imply, even in the absence of a specific statement, that such names are exempt from the relevant protective laws and regulations and therefore free for general use.
The publisher, the authors and the editors are safe to assume that the advice and information in this book are believed to be true and accurate at the date of publication. Neither the publisher nor the authors or the editors give a warranty, express or implied, with respect to the material contained herein or for any errors or omissions that may have been made. The publisher remains neutral with regard to jurisdictional claims in published maps and institutional affiliations.

Cover illustration: Fatima Jamadar

Printed on acid-free paper

This Palgrave Macmillan imprint is published by Springer Nature
The registered company is Macmillan Publishers Ltd.
The registered company address is: The Campus, 4 Crinan Street, London, N1 9XW, United Kingdom

Preface

This book is the outcome of our work together on the topic of chronic pain. Our research, *Communicating Chronic Pain: Interdisciplinary Strategies for Non-Textual Data*, aimed to explore non-textual methods of communicating about pain, on social media and through arts workshops, to find ways to enable pain sufferers to communicate about pain in ways that did not rely on language, and to develop methods for analysis of these expressions. It did this through an exploration of chronic pain expressions on social media sites such as Flickr and Tumblr, and a series of arts workshops exploring drawing, painting, and sculpting; digital photography; sound and music; and physical theatre. More information and outputs from the workshops can be found on the project's website, http://www.communicatingchronicpain.org/.

This edited volume was prompted by the project's final conference, *Communicating Chronic Pain: Creative Approaches, Interdisciplinary Frameworks*, held on 18 September 2014. A number of presenters from that conference are included in this volume, including Lucy Bending, Sarah Goldingay, and Sue Ziebland. Deborah Padfield and Jude Rosen spoke at an event we organised around chronic pain and arts-based approaches at the LSE Literary Festival in 2015. We would like to acknowledge that there were people who contributed to the conference and the research who for a number of reasons could not be part of the final volume, but who nevertheless also shaped it, including Ulises

Moreno-Tabarez, Yasmin Gunaratnam, and Lisa Folkmarsson Käll. As the book project progressed, we were very fortunate to be able to draw in additional perspectives including those of Rebeca Pardo and Montse Morcate, Alice Andrews, and Trish O'Shea and colleagues, all of which, we believe, strengthen the volume with interdisciplinary and collaborative approaches.

Painscapes aims to provide alternative ways of understanding pain, through devices such as images, poems, historical texts, stories, and qualitative interviews. Our aim has been to bring these perspectives together as modes of understanding which both intersect and diverge, helping us to navigate pain's complexities. This book draws together perspectives from sociology, the medical sciences and anthropology; visual art, particularly photography; literature and theatre. Throughout, the goal has been to engage with these perspectives without privileging any one single standpoint.

Communicating Chronic Pain was supported by the UK's Economic and Social Research Council via the National Centre for Research Methods under the Methodological Innovations Projects scheme (Grant number DU/512589108). We remain very grateful to the workshop leaders and participants who shared their ideas and experiences with us. Our research would not have been the same without our co-investigators on the *Communicating Chronic Pain* project, Flora Cornish and Aude Bicquelet. We also extend thanks to Ricardo Carvalho and Lutz Issler, who were essential interlocutors throughout the research process. The *Communicating Chronic Pain* project benefitted from the support of our advisory board members Amanda Williams, Mick Thacker, Deborah Padfield, Kate Jolly, Charles Pither, and Beverly Collett, and we are grateful for their involvement.

London, UK	EJ Gonzalez-Polledo
London, UK	Jen Tarr
May 2017	

Contents

1 **Painscapes** 1
  EJ Gonzalez-Polledo

2 **'The Sad Language of Pain': S. Weir Mitchell,
  the American Civil War, and Interpreting
  Physical Suffering** 25
  Lucy Bending

3 **An Essay on the Space Outside Pain Where
  the Poem Takes Place** 41
  Jude Rosen

4 **Act Like It Hurts: Questions of Role and Authenticity
  in the Communication of Chronic Pain** 61
  Sarah Goldingay

5 **Articulating Pain: Writing the Autoimmune Self** 83
  Alice Andrews

6 Exhibiting Pain, Death and Grief: From the Art Gallery
   to the Image Shared Online   107
   Montse Morcate

7 Pain and the Internet: Transforming the Experience?   129
   Nikki Newhouse, Helen Atherton, and Sue Ziebland

8 Photography and Mental Illness: Feeding or Combating
   the Stigma of Invisible Pain Online and Offline   157
   Rebeca Pardo

9 ADJOIN   183
   Trish O'Shea, Mark Wilkinson, and Jackie Jones

10 Face2face: Sharing the Photograph Within Medical Pain
   Encounters—A Means of Democratisation   205
   Deborah Padfield and Joanna M. Zakrzewska

11 Painscapes and Method   229
   Jen Tarr

Index   249

List of Figures

Fig. 9.1	Collection by Trish O'Shea	187
Fig. 9.2	Sample by Trish O'Shea	191
Fig. 9.3	Tower of strength by Trish O'Shea	192
Fig. 9.4	Restriction by Trish O'Shea	193
Fig. 9.5	Pain relief by Trish O'Shea	196
Fig. 9.6	Confidential, by Trish O'Shea and Jackie Jones	199
Fig. 9.7	Detail of confidential by Trish O'Shea and Jackie Jones	200
Fig. 9.8	Detail of confidential, by Trish O'Shea and Jackie Jones	201
Fig. 9.9	Detail of confidential by Trish O'Shea and Jackie Jones	202
Fig. 10.1	Image of pain co-created by Deborah Padfield with Liz Aldous from the series *face2face*, 2008–2013 © Deborah Padfield	214
Fig. 10.2	Image of pain co-created by Deborah Padfield with Chandrakant Khoda from the series *face2face*, 2008–2013 © Deborah Padfield	215
Fig. 10.3	Image of pain co-created by Deborah Padfield with Alison Glenn from the series *face2face*, 2008–2013 © Deborah Padfield	217

Fig. 10.4 Image of pain co-created by Deborah Padfield with
John Pates from the series *perceptions of pain*,
2001–2006 © Deborah Padfield Reproduced by kind
permission of Dewi Lewis Publishing   218

Fig. 10.5 Image of pain co-created by Deborah Padfield with
Yante from the series *face2face*, 2008–2013 ©
Deborah Padfield   220

1

Painscapes

EJ Gonzalez-Polledo

Pain is imbricated in clinical and experimental histories where the transformation of subjective experience into scientific measure was a form of political physiology.[1] Tracing a history of pain in medicine, Joanna Bourke notes that the application of ether substances in surgical pain relief for surgical applications was not until 50 years after the discovery of this substance, as its widespread use was intertwined with Romantic preoccupations about the democratic distribution of happiness that pushed the pain relief agenda as a legitimate goal during the Enlightenment. Davy's discovery of ether was framed by vitalist concerns about the effect of an under-stimulating gas vis-à-vis pain as an over-stimulant, both seen to put patients at risk.[2] As it became possible to render a person insensible to pain while keeping them alive, the principle of application of pain relief was grounded in forms of calculation of preferable suffering. Pernick's history of anaesthesia demonstrates that the application of pain relief relied on the acceptance of suffering ratios and probabilities of death, and that the 'utilitarian professionalism' that guided the early

EJ Gonzalez-Polledo (✉)
Department of Anthropology Goldsmiths, University of London, London, UK

development of anaesthetics was itself rooted in physicians' 'search for a moderate consensus ideology'[3] that would allow them to bridge disciplinary cleavages. Choices between maintaining life and alleviating pain were affectively grounded, as physicians understood their professional duty as 'demanding the unhesitating infliction of extreme suffering in order to save lives'.[4] Social position, race, and gender and age played a major role in this form of calculus, effectively determining who would and would not receive anaesthetics, and to what degree. In some instances, pain was seen as a positive experience that could be beneficial. Physicians counted in their duties to 'bolster the courage of patients',[5] seeking to actively 'develop' their moral qualities through pain management. In contrast, patients were dismissed as responding emotionally while under the influence of anaesthetics, and the encounters between practitioners and patients were seen as dangerous even for practitioners, as the application of anaesthetics was perceived to threaten the social, sometimes also the sexual order between patients and their clinicians. Indeed, as Bourke argues, the development of anaesthesia was enmeshed in wartime logics and logistics, practical barriers that determined the availability of pain relief remedies, as well as defective equipment and incomplete medical training that added up to unequal pain relief provision, grounded in moral anxieties and spiritual dangers.[6]

Turning pain into an object of medical study 'involved separating clinical pain from laboratory pain, and most importantly, separating chronic pain from acute pain'.[7] The history of anaesthetics is based on instrumental correlations that attest to the reality of pain, based on certainties such as the fact that 'a small prick with a needle in the finger causes tolerable pain, whereas a strong blow with a hammer to the same place normally unleashes severe pain'.[8] Correlational measures of pain and tissue damage were predicated on assumptions about the stability of pain as an object of investigation, privileging purely mechanical values of sensation as data since these produced replicable results. Although judgements such as these provided pain with unique characteristics, and its status as research object,[9] these same judgements imbued chronic pain with a problematic status: not only is it a private experience to which no one but the person in pain has direct access, but it resists medical actions and explanations in its persistence. As social, emotional, and psychological domains are brought to bear on the aetiology and definition of pain, clinical research has progressively veered away from early theories of pain that followed the Cartesian model of an isomorphic relation between pain and tissue injury.[10] Yet, as Goldberg has noted, pain without lesion became an object of consistent epistemic stigmatisation in clinical research and practice well into the twenty first century, supported by the rise of a culture of mechanical objectivity and evidence-based practice and backed by historic paradigmatic court rulings.[11]

Definitions of chronic pain have been notoriously difficult to standardise.[12] The long-term effects of chronic pain do not easily map onto prognostic values and indicators.[13] Biomedical health narratives imagined pain through metaphors of survival which depend on the recognition and elimination of pain. Contraposing the pain-free body to the body afflicted by pain, pain is seen to trigger a form of warfare,[14] calling for action-oriented technical responses to tackle its effects and for long-term adaptive approaches to healing. Indeed, 'a good life' should not be painful or difficult, nor lived through the kind of alienated senses of subjectivity and relationality that often arise from anomalous long-term pain.[15] However, although ubiquitous forms of pain transverse religious, cultural, and historical boundaries,[16] social scientists have long known that pain derived from long-term illness is not universal, and neither are its effects.[17] Persistent pain is, rather, anomic,[18] escaping systematisation in a coherent system of meanings or values. Pain may be an event of total loss that fractures any and all notions of totality.[19] It may be a fluid state across patterns of flare and remittance in which, alongside the endurance of pain itself, there is an inability to restore levels of function held prior to pain's inception.

Thinking through emotional and communicational aspects as critical to pain experience, Bendelow and Williams argue for an approach to pain beyond models focused on sensation and based on the Cartesian split between body and mind.[20] Against the medicalised view, Bendelow and Williams recast pain as an experience of being in the world, irreducible to the qualities of sensation, and grounded in communication processes at the intersection between biology and culture. Pain extends beyond individual bodies to inhabit practices, relations of care, regulations, pharmacokinetics and multiple, partially connected practice cultures that normalise notions of health and ability, producing pain no longer only as sensation, but as an epistemological, social, and political ecology. People who live with pain long term trace their pain to personal experiences of misdiagnosis, stigma, and undertreatment, to the extent that, analysing the global patterns that make chronic pain endemic, Manderson and Smith-Morris argue that 'increasingly, chronic, long-term conditions are not naturally occurring ones, but are those for which the political will and economic resources are simply not brought to bear for a given community'.[21] As the prevalence of chronic conditions becomes an increasingly ubiquitous global public health concern,[22] the increased prevalence of chronic pain is linked to factors shaping access to resources, socioeconomic status, stress at work, occupational status, race, and education, locating pain across relations between policy and politics. Correlations between pain and disability highlight, furthermore, that feeling pain and being in pain are not co-terminous. People with lower incomes are not only more likely to be more disabled by pain, but research demonstrates that there is a relation between social conditions and the intensification of pain.[23] For Wilkinson and Kleinman, social suffering is now an extension of illness made routine in everyday life by the force of stigma, material deprivation, and compounding forms of epistemic, medical, and political injustice.[24]

In this context, new questions are emerging across academic disciplines about the relation between pain experience and pain expression, which point to complex entanglements between pain epistemologies, the justification and provision of healthcare services, and the dynamics of clinical protocols in lives where pain is present. Addressing pain communication, from this perspective, requires an ongoing dialogue between the humanities, art, philosophy, and the social and biomedical sciences. Combining insights from anthropology, sociology, the medical humanities, and the arts, this volume draws on phenomenological and post-phenomenological approaches to pain communication to enquire about the devices, methods, and artefacts through which pain is known and lived. It focuses on the material, informational, and practical worlds that emerge as pain is made social, and how the endurance of these worlds, their disruptions, and transformative potential pose new questions about the epistemologies and transactional politics of pain and method. Using multiple devices such as stories, poetry, photographs, concepts, and relational aesthetics, contributors reimagine pain through intersubjective, temporal, and material and knowledge ecologies, *painscapes*. These configurations are meant to be totalising representations of pain experience but map the complexity of pain across physical, social, and intersubjective domains, following key concepts, objects, and methods to conceptualise the ways of knowing, relating, and dwelling that resonate in everyday experiences of pain.

Pain and/*as* Communication

Pain literature in the humanities insistently recounts pain's resistance to language. For Wittgenstein, in Philosophical Investigations,[25] language holds an ambivalent potential, as it betrays the inherently private nature of pain, which makes language liable of misrepresenting pain, at the same language is an extension of pain, makes pain public. Elaine Scarry has clearly illustrated that the experience of pain and language relates only partially. 'Physical pain', she writes, '-unlike any other state of consciousness- has no referential content. It is not "of" or "for" anything'.[26] Scarry argues that the indeterminate location and immersive experience of pain bring about a state prior to language, arguing, against currency of biomedical knowledge, that only those who are not in pain can become the reliable narrators of pain experience. Arthur Frank's work on illness narratives demonstrated how the relation between bodies and narrative reflects both cultural ideals and ethical choices, since, ultimately, through narrative, the body is the moral problem addressed in narratives of self-making.[27] A growing body of literature in the fields of medical humanities and narrative medicine has come to revalue narrative as a transformative device in clinical contexts and beyond.[28] Drawing on Eve K Sedgwick's notion, Jurecic reflects on the value of illness narratives as 'reparative reading'.[29] Exploring the role of illness in professional writers' accounts, Jurecic argues traces a parallel between the emergence of narratives about illness and a new role of everyday experience in literary practice. In the nineteenth century, memoirs by clinicians and their heroic narratives of discovery preceded first-person narratives of illness. Unlike full autobiographies, these narratives were rather 'sanatorium narratives',[30] chronicling an encounter with illness, with medical staff, or with other patients. But as changes in the patient–doctor relationships became pronounced after the 1950s, and then again after population health crises such as the HIV/AIDS, the quest of meaning in illness proliferated in multiple genres. Straddling between the noble act of testimony and the impossible task of speaking about trauma, medical, and public engagement with these narratives produced qualitative changes in how individuals faced illness.[31] Jurecic argues that illness narratives generate productive tensions at interstices, taking from illness narratives their capacity to multiply the presence of illness, to speak 'out of what spaces I may speak of it, or be spoken for' as Sedgwick put it, a place where it is possible to point towards instability and uncertainty. Consider Lochlann Jain's definition of 'living in prognosis',[32] which develops a sense that cancer diagnosis, repeatedly deferred and warped by cognitive dissonances between a lived sense of vitality and a personal sense of cancer imminence, and the 'objective' statistical accounts of symptoms brought forward by medical professionals with no direct experience of cancer. Jain was presented with a calculative process based on probabilities of effectivity of particular treatments. Numbers and statistics waged as a measure of real chances of survival were intentionally devoid of politics, yet measured the politics of knowledge against the process of living. Jain writes that 'the statistics that offer the promise of beating the odds also evacuate the politics of prognoses'.[33] Indeed, being treated as a statistic observation not only clashed with Jain's sense of embodiment, selfhood and aspiration in the diagnostic process, but with her actual progress once a treatment course was approved.[34] Living in prognosis suspended the sense of passing time, and of temporal frameworks such as age, generation, illness stage and lifespan. Jain's testimony attests to how consequences of ineffective or injurious ways of knowing treatment had real consequences, affecting some survivors more than illness itself.

Informational worlds are key to the making of everyday pain and disability worlds.[35] Living in pain implies reinterpretation of what a normal life can be like,[36] as of pain temporalities overlap with poverty, normal practices of care and neglect, imbricating the experience of social and physical pain with social dynamics of care and the failings of bureaucratic and administrative systems. Lauren Berlant offers a compelling reading of their entanglement in the Dardennes Brothers film *Rosetta* (1999),[37] which chronicles the devastating physical effects of social pain through the protagonist's impossible quest for aspirational normativity. For Berlant, the indistinction between physical and 'political, economic and affective forms of existence' relates broad kinds of social dynamics to a critical interrogation of the place of pain in the making of political worlds.[38] From this perspective, pain becomes an environment, rather than an object, whose knowledges, practices and artefacts are, as Berlant suggested, 'themselves normatively mediated'.[39] For example, ethnographic studies of pain management[40] evince how dominant ways of knowing pain affect how pain is perceived. Anthropologist Jean Jackson has argued that distinctions between experiences of pain, the emotional states that come with it, and pain behaviours is ambivalent, and the credibility of self-reports of pain can diminish over time. Cultural or collective meanings of illness can work counterintuitively to delegitimise certain forms of pain experience, which are understood as 'meaningless', lacking cultural appraisal or contestation.[41] Jackson's study focused on how interactions at a pain clinic, characterised by a disconnection between patient reports and medical terminology, suggest that forms of address actually impact the perceived reality of pain, its nature, and the perceived responsibilities associated with stigma. During the course of one year, Jackson developed a methodology of 'cognitive restructuring' to track how changes in how pain was thought correlated with self-reports of pain improvement. At this clinic, 'real pain' became notoriously difficult to standardise. While it was agreed that pain 'performed a function' in most cases, whether the nature of this function could be considered authentic was routinely made an object of contention. Jackson reports that "clinicians' understandings of pain are complex and varied, depending on their medical specialty and on the specifics of a given case (…) the clinicians' debate focuses on the extent to which chronic pain is due to psychogenic, rather than physical aspects, causes, and the consequent implications for treatment'.[42] Indeed, the focus on pain's aetiology derived a distinction between 'real' pain—organic, and pain for which the patient is not responsible and 'unreal' pain—involving somatisation and possible gains for the patient, such as access to medication or an assumed ability to derive social gains from 'performing' pain. Combinations of 'real' and 'unreal' pain were the most common for patients. For Jackson, patients were 'placed on a bind: on one hand, some hope is being offered in the form of pain relief, on the other, the suggestion is clear that their notions about their own pain are wrong'.[43] Compounding the notion that unreal pain can be willed away by psychological therapy or non-medical therapies has far reaching implications, as patients began to resist the pain clinic's message because it was seen to perpetuate stigma. Jackson, therefore, became suspicious that self-reports of improvement—that were used to compile improvement indices—reflected actual improvement. Rather, her ethnography suggests that patients routinely changed their understanding of pain, and how they communicated about it, as their own pain measures were broken down and rewritten over the course of the programme to fit with the clinic's prognostic indicators.

The importance of illness narratives, from this perspective, would not least be the capacity of the story to be read, and of a reader to construct the time-bound causal patterns that relate sense-making to primary experience. Placing a teller and a reader at the centre of a narrative process highlights how stark objectivity may not be possible in the realm of human interactions. For Morris,[44] fiction provides a bedrock for a 'postmodern' illness model, understood beyond dualistic, mechanistic, and reductive definitions of body versus mind. At the crossroads of biology and culture, this new approach 'acknowledges the emergence of powerful cultural forces from mass media and government subsidies to multinational drug companies', revealing 'how illness can be crucially modified or wholly reconstructed by its contact with narrative'.[45] For Morris, the implications of the clash between individual and cultural narratives are primarily ethical. Indeed, a narrative ethics must be willing to pose difficult to answer questions about intended and unintended damage to patients, and to face up to the challenge narrative's potential to challenge the decidability of knowledge. For example, in an autoethnographic study of fibromyalgia, Greenhalgh highlights how chronic pain objects, materials and devices have social lives of their own. They can produce disability as an administrative category with recourse to particular policies and regulations,[46] even though, rather than on a physical basis, it depends on social judgements of normalcy, and the measuring of bodies and everyday realities against ideals that characterises disability worlds.[47]

In Greenhalgh's process of being misdiagnosed with fibromyalgia, pain, like disability, was normalised through undemocratic access to technology and the materialities and politics of communication processes. In clinical encounters, her identity was transformed from that of a 'person with arthritis' to a 'fibromyalgic-arthritic patient', a process that involved normalising symptoms and undergoing a course of treatment as part of an erroneous diagnosis.[48] For Greenhalgh, discourses of truth masked as scientific and value neutral put the patient in jeopardy particularly when the complex and chaotic reality of the clinical encounter is denied. However, rather than accept epistemic injustice as an inevitable outcome of clinical relations, a phenomenological and postbiomedical notion of illness must be crucially concerned with values and politics of communication.[49] Greenhalgh calls the doctor's account of the patients' ills a story which draws attention to the moving boundaries between fact and fiction.[50] As a pragmatic tool, narrative can displace questions about who is right or wrong in composing a problem. Crucially, Morris argues, narrative would force medicine 'to confront the recognition that pain is not just a medical or neurological problem but implacably biocultural'.[51] In these sense, illness narratives stage a cultural politics of emotion. Morris draws these politics around encounters 'in the hallway', encounters deeply entrenched in personal experiences of illness that produce new critical agenda for bioethics.[52] Such a programme as this can intentionally replace the ethics of good and evil which hides behind bureaucratic bodies and institutional decisions, linking cultural narratives back to both identities and everyday moralities of the people for whom they matter.

In this context, pain communication becomes a key site of enquiry. Through communication, like illness, as Carel perceptively proposes, can be a phenomenological notion in contrast with the naturalistic definition that accounts primarily for physical fact, it is 'objective (and objectifying), neutral and third-personal'.[53] Carel's first-person-centred epistemology is the basis of a shift to abandon the framework of pathology and bring forward new questions about the social, cultural, epistemological determinants of illness.[54] But more crucially, a focus on communication can become a key site to develop ethical forms of communication concerned with identifying the structures that underpin experience, while taking difference seriously and recognising that others' experiences may be incommensurable.[55] For Carel and Kidd, this process

> involves a transition from an "informational perspective" which sees the speaker as a "potential recipient or source of information" to the 'participant perspective', in which we see the quest for knowledge as a shared enterprise and the patient speaker as "competent to carry out some particular activity that has a fundamental role in carrying out inquiries[56]

Reflecting on clinical experience, Biro has described how a creative practice of listening could transform the clinical encounter with people who 'try to find the right words, but typically come up empty'.[57] It is perhaps the difficulty of finding the right words, he argues, that has tipped clinical assessments of pain from relying on technical assessment protocols, such as the McGill Pain Questionnaire, to instead provide people seeking pain services a basic series of pictures known as the faces pain scale.[58] Biro argues, however, that transcending literal linguistic representations may help clinicians get better at identifying and treating pain. While the rich vocabulary involved in metaphorising the action of pain of the McGill Pain questionnaire goes a long way in making pain representable through language, the simplicity of the faces scale, using pre-linguistic expression, makes it possible to communicate in practice. As Nancy has noted, while hearing has multiple meanings organised through different combinations of tension, intention and attention, listening, on the other hand, evolves around the word 'entendre', which is linked to 'comprendre'—'understanding'.[59] To listen, unlike hearing, does not relate to sensation but seeks to achieve a presence in the 'resonance of a return'.[60] Through listening, a listener opens to the world a field of relational ethics.[61]

Biro's patients spoke of living across two worlds, a sense that the depth and elusive presence of pain is indistinguishable from its significance. Here the metaphorical and contextual nature of pain communication becomes a crucial site of enquiry where new questions about the relational and ecological form of pain can be formulated, drawing on the ways in which different media can draw multiple emotional, aesthetic, political and sublime responses, and not, like in language, directly through it.[62]

Painscapes

This volume aims to interrogate intersections between pain and communication to ascertain in what contexts and to what effects pain becomes known.[63] Much like Veena Das' methods compose the problem of pain from a vernacular,[64] the chapters in this collection present a series of contexts as 'scenes of instruction', presenting particular assemblages of media, context, and critique as key interfaces of ordinary ethics. Advocating a descent into ordinary practice, cultivating the sensibilities of the everyday.[65] In a broad cultural discussion of modernity, Arjun Appadurai argued that the suffix—scape captured a new role of imagination in social life. Not only that the tensions between cultural homogenisation and heterogenisation demanded a dynamic framework 'where an array of empirical facts could be brought to bear on [the] argument', but a sense that theoretical tools, even models and flexible theories, come short of addressing the complexity of global cultural flows. The suffix—scape, as Arjun Appadurai (1996) proposed to understand it, brings into relationship multiple dimensions of complex phenomena, describing landscapes which may be fluid and irregular, and which do not take an objective form from every point of view. Rather, painscapes are perspectival constructs, inflected by the situatedness of multiple actors, who form part of other landscapes, and who both constitute and experience these landscapes in the process of imagining their capacities and shortcomings.

Imagining painscapes brings contributors to map socio-material formations connected with ways of knowing pain, refracting pain through the lines that entangle medical, psychosocial and political domains of pain experience. Navigating these domains opens up a transsensible space that brings into focus transits and exchanges between multiple modalities of perception and technologies of capture in the making of pain worlds. Focusing on the multiple *relations* between experience and expression brings forward a practice of witnessing that takes pain beyond the dominant visualism paradigm in philosophy and in science, bearing witness in ways that exceed vision: just as there is no eyelid to protect from hearing, sound demands to be brought into experience in ways that surrender attention and elicit an affective, conceptual and emotional response. Critical to this new focus on pain communication, then, is the notion of attunement as a critical outcome of communication. This notion brings to a relation context, media and message, and it calls into question the idea that communication must aim to generalise experience, seeking, instead, a capacity to sense, figure, amplify, attend, sensitise, and translate the complexity of the material forces that structure sensation. Tone and tendency are fundamental to the transformation of physical qualities into working concepts, since connecting thinking and feeling foregrounds the critical role of the encounter as a generative, not representative time-space.[66] Crossing human and non-human boundaries, attunement involves locking in qualities, frequencies and vibrations in a communicative event, and connecting capacities of perception to capacities of understanding and intervention, involving the elements assembled in the process of communication.

Bending opens the collection by reflecting on the historical underpinnings of the difficulty of communicating pain. Focusing on the American Civil war, Bending follows the claims to pain's incommunicability to Army Assistant Surgeon J.J Woodward and army doctor Silas Weir Mitchell, who observed that it is only when a person *performs* pain, by verbally admitting to its existence, that the *foreignness* of pain, its signs and symptoms, can be translated. Focusing on how these doctors learnt to listen to 'the sad language of pain', Bending opens up the power of language, and its limitations, to translate 'real' pain worlds. Mitchell advocated a professionalisation of pain medicine not only as a means of recognising the unprecedented forms of pain soldiers encountered during the war but also of grappling with entanglements of word and symptom—real and imagined—as well as with their social and emotional effects. Bending chronicles how in this period, *seeing* pain, rather than *listening to* pain, became the gold standard of diagnostic procedures, constructing the ways in which the 'compelling, more truthful' character of the body's somatic responses was preferred over words by doctors, until it is the doctor himself who is doubted in his capacity to accurately translate pain. For Bending, Mitchell's story brings pain back into moral sets of relationships, and the practical historicity that provides symptoms truth value to ways of knowing in scientific and clinical relations. At the other end of this story, the presence and immediacy of a Crohn's disease diagnosis, Rosen newly engages history and poetry to bear on her experience of chronic pain. Using poems as devices that connect temporalities of pain and clinical pain cultures, Rosen casts the practice of writing as a generative form of resistance to cultural debilitating narratives of chronic pain, using writing to open up in between spaces where people, organs, and drugs, social living and cultural representations share a common temporality. Rosen strings these temporal thresholds through the long persistent temporalities of chronic pain, mirroring memory through the momentous difference of poetic effect, and marking the space of writing as a space of transformation 'outside' of pain. Entangled in this space, writing and sensation unfold multiple tensions between pain and identity, intentionality and indeterminacy, creativity and rupture. The point of pain, Rosen speculates, might be to let the interface of a poem extend the political boundaries of the body beyond the self, in the process making 'the unbearable funny, and hence, bearable'.

Challenging clear-cut binaries between subjective and structural forces, public and private domains, the performance of pain is bound by the recognition of authenticity. Goldingay delves into the mutually constitutive roles of performing doctors and patients in chronic pain related clinical encounters. Her chapter interrogates the cultural fragility associated with the figure of chronic pain patients as they approach the clinical environment, and particularly, the contrast that emerges between this fragility and the coping strategies a person in pain necessarily deploys in everyday living. Goldingay analyses the medical encounter to tease out the expectations, procedures, and experiences that compose patient and doctor roles in the chronic pain drama. Drawing on the inherent dynamism of these roles, and their reliance on conflict, Goldingay unpacks how medical training and performance afford particular cultural constructions of both pain and patient roles, and how, inverting doctor–patient roles and taking non-verbal communication seriously when interpreting pain communication might deeply destabilise the epistemological structures of pain. Taking pain further beyond the limits of modern subjectivity through a reading of autoimmunity, Andrews draws on a close reading of Derrida's philosophy as well as cybernetics to conceptualise autoimmunity. Although autoimmunity refers to self-infliction by etymology, Andrews rethinks this notion in connections across biomedical, political, and philosophical realms. Autoimmunity is at the heart of the modern paradox that understands the self in opposition to a hostile environment. Radically reworking the connections that engineer the I, the authority of scientific discourses, one's autobiography, and healthcare system, Andrews undoes the gap between 'the one who writes and the one who is written', the autonomous one and the one who is 'marked violently, painfully, by that which "one" is not'. Following the logic of autoimmunity, its endurance and destructive quest, Andrews proposes a deconstructive move that focuses directly on pain as a double bind, 'where one is not only put in question but is put to the question'. Andrews offers a new lexicon to navigate pain as an aporia, which produces, at the same time, pain as a form of communication and the information pathways of self-creation. Autoimmunity, from this point of view, is based on a contradiction, which, in Andrews' words 'is just as likely to maintain a system as it is to deconstruct it'.

Interrogating the theme of pain's visibility in popular culture, Morcate explores how experiences of pain confront us with an existential abyss that destabilises notions of truth and presence, since it is only in an effort of remembering and communicating that pain is given form. The artworks she presents instantiate the past to engender multiple futurities—a practice of listening to images' resonances to tune in to what has not been said.[67] Sensing worlds through and beyond the site-specificity of artworks leads Morcate to conceptualise the role artworks might play as vehicles of grief. Morcate tracks significant shifts in pain art worlds around changes in conventional representations of pain across the twentieth century, fuelled by changes in biomedicine and by the rise of photography as a medium to explore life and death. Morcate explores artworks where the quality of detachment—between artist and pain—provides an almost analytic approach to pain, as well as a new political way into pain. By opening up pain controversies, and detaching pain from the individual experience of suffering, these artworks expose often-patronising cultural discourses of pain, particularly at a time when digital technologies and social media platforms have made it possible for artists to develop new contexts and media forms to communicate about pain, newly involving publics and media in feedback loops that transform both pain experience and expression.

As pain communication finds its way into public, networked spaces, shared ordinary experiences of pain become powerful connective and transformative interventions. Newhouse, Atherton, and Ziebland track pain communication in social media platforms and online forums. Their contribution follows how chronic pain patients in these platforms have become health prosumers—active contributors to the production of health communication as well as informed consumers. Using online worlds to find experiential information, these internet users find new ways of understanding their condition, and develop and maintain supportive relations that have a direct effect in how they live with pain. Further, these platforms are significantly transforming interfaces of exchange between clinicians and patients. The key to understanding the success of these platforms, particularly their capacity to transform experiences of pain, lies in the capacity of storytelling—a process of making visible that exposes pain communication beyond factual biomedical language. Yet the increased visibility of chronic pain online, as Pardo perceptively argues in her contribution, can also become a vehicle for stigmatising some forms of chronic pain, particularly those deriving from mental health conditions. Pardo recasts the stigma of invisible pain by interrogating the role of photography and photojournalism in social perception of illness and pain. Using photographic media to call into question the objectivity of scientific pain images, Pardo approaches photographic practices as systems that connect artists, users, and issues through culturally specific aesthetic and moral frameworks, articulating around themselves real and imagined practices and communities. While early in the medical history of pain, photographs classified mental illness traits and symptoms, clinical photography focusing on literal representations of individual conditions became the standard for the representation of mental illness, yet failed to make pain related to mental health visible. Later, approaches in photojournalism followed the critical voices in psychiatry and the social sciences to contest these representations through critical, often highly social images where the photographer's neutrality was radically called into question. The current shift towards online sharing of pain images, mixing self-referential and critical accounts, points to a gradual shift towards a 'domestication' and democratisation of pain images, signalling the beginning of new ways of communicating about pain in ever growing series published in platforms that offered more control and ethical sharing options to users.

The last three chapters reflect on the relation between pain and representation through the perspective of practice. These chapters illuminate aspects of pain that highlight the need to develop a post-phenomenological framework, concerned with the experience of pain in contexts of practice.[68] Thinking through the practice of listening, O'Shea, Wilkinson, and Jones present the results of Adjoin, a collaborative project that brought them to reflect on the experience of living with arthritis. Using photography to explore the experience of pain and to share it in the clinical encounter with Wilkinson, O'Shea reflects on how the practice of photographing, O'Shea's art project brings collected images, dialogues, reflections, and information resonances to constitute the experience of pain as itself multiple, anchored in the juxtaposition of scales, instruments, technologies of representation, the kinds of knowledge, identities, and patient journeys they afford. While O'Shea asks how the language of pain may be depicted and presented to others, Padfield and Zarkrzewska interrogate the potential of images in clinical consultations to improve diagnostic outcomes. Padfield and Zarkrzewska demonstrate how the mechanic specificities of the photographic medium might be particularly suited to be deployed in chronic pain consultations, making the experience of pain present in the consultation room, visible and actionable. Advocating a broad definition of pain across biomarkers and emotional and social pain domains, Padfield and Zarkrzewska present an integrative approach that brings to the fore the inherently narrative character of medicine. Not only do images facilitate doctor–patient dialogue allowing patients to communicate pain in a language of their choice, but working with pain patients at different stages of their journey can help people living with long-term conditions break away with the paralysis that is often experienced as a result of pain. Padfield and Zarkrzewska demonstrate how through a co-creative process, participants in their research were able to project a plastic image of identity, where the practices of observation, witness, and analysis were key to developing new understandings of identities of people living in long-term pain as flexible rather than static.

Finally, Tarr's conclusion brings into focus the relation between pain and method. Drawing on research across a range of projects, Tarr demonstrates the multiple capacities of method to generate pain as a multiple reality. As a mode of addressing pain's shifting constitution, marked by perspective as it is by knowing practices and imagination, Tarr frames painscapes as assemblages that work through the productive and limiting capacities of method—methods that tease out and enclose, reify and reveal, and ultimately produce the contrasts, transferences, and dialogues needed to compose the problem of pain.

Notes

1. Cf. Meloni, Maurizio. *Political Biology: Science and Social Values in Human Heredity from Eugenics to Epigenetics* (Basingstoke, Hampshire; New York, NY: Palgrave Macmillan, 2016).
2. Bourke, Joanna. *The Story of Pain: From Prayer to Painkillers* (New York, NY: Oxford University Press, 2014), 282.
3. Pernick, Martin S. *A Calculus of Suffering: Pain, Professionalism, and Anesthesia in Nineteenth-Century America* (New York: Columbia University Press, 1985), 105.
4. Pernick, *A Calculus of Suffering*, 109.
5. Ibid., 288.
6. Bourke, *The Story of Pain*, 285.
7. Baszanger, *Inventing Pain Medicine*, 2.
8. Moscoso, Javier. *Pain: A Cultural History* (Basingstoke: Palgrave Macmillan, 2012), 173.
9. Baszanger, Isabelle. *Inventing Pain Medicine: From the Laboratory to the Clinic* (New Brunswick, NJ; London: Rutgers University Press, 1998).
10. The biopsychosocial model of pain, the gold standard of pain diagnosis, proposes a heuristic model of the interrelation between biological, psychological, and social and cultural factors. See Gatchel, Robert J., Yuan Bo Peng, Madelon L. Peters, Perry N. Fuchs, and Dennis C. Turk. "The Biopsychosocial Approach to Chronic Pain: Scientific Advances and Future Directions". *Psychological Bulletin* 133, no. 4 (2007: 581–624). Gate control theories such as the allostatic load hypothesis situate social environments as determinants at the core of not only pain prevalence, but thresholds of pain mortality. Brunner, E., and M. Marmot. "Social

Organization, Stress, and Health". In *Social Determinants of Health*, edited by M. Marmot and R. G. Wilkinson (New York: Oxford University Press, 2006); Borrell, L. N., and N. Nguyen. "Racial/Ethnic Disparities in All-Cause Mortality in U.S. Adults: The Effect of Allostatic Load". *Public Health Reports* 125 (2010); and Torrance, N., A. M. Elliott, A. J. Lee, and B. H. Smith. "Severe Chronic Pain Is Associated with Increased 10 Year Mortality. A Cohort Record Linkage Study". *European Journal of Pain* 14, no. 4 (Apr. 2010): 380–386.
11. Goldberg, Daniel S. "Pain, Objectivity and History: Understanding Pain Stigma". *Medical Humanities* (2017).
12. Though there have been multiple attempts at standardising the definition of chronic pain, see, for instance, Ruan, Xiulu, and Alan David Kaye. "Defining Chronic Pain". *The Journal of Rheumatology* 43, no. 4 (2016): 826–827. In clinical research, standardisation can sometimes be viewed with suspicion; see Sullivan, Mark D., Alex Cahana, Stuart Derbyshire, and John D. Loeser. "What Does It Mean to Call Chronic Pain a Brain Disease?" *The Journal of Pain* 14, no. 4: 317–322.
13. Manderson, Lenore. *Surface Tensions: Surgery, Bodily Boundaries, and the Social Self* (Walnut Creek, CA: Left Coast Press, 2011).
14. See Martin, Emily. *Flexible Bodies: Tracking Immunity in American Culture from the Days of Polio to the Age of Aids* (Boston: Beacon Press, 1994); also Biro, David. *Listening to Pain: Finding Words, Compassion, and Relief* (New York; London: W.W. Norton, 2011).
15. Arney, William Ray, and Bernard J. Bergen. "The Anomaly, the Chronic Patient and the Play of Medical Power". *Sociology of Health & Illness* 5, no. 1 (1983): 1–24.
16. Coakley, Sarah, and Kay Kaufman Shelemay. *Pain and Its Transformations: The Interface of Biology and Culture* (Cambridge, MA; London: Harvard University Press, 2007).
17. Kleinman, Arthur, Paul Brodwin, Byron Good, and Mary-Jo DelVecchio Good. "Pain as Human Experience: An Introduction". In *Pain as Human Experience: An Anthropological Perspective*, edited by Arthur Kleinman, Paul Brodwin, Byron Good, and Mary-Jo DelVecchio Good (Berkeley: University of California Press, 1992).
18. Hilbert, Richard A. "The Acultural Dimensions of Chronic Pain: Flawed Reality Construction and the Problem of Meaning". *Social Problems* 31, no. 4 (1984): 365–378.

19. Eng, David L., and David Kazanjian. *Loss: The Politics of Mourning* (Berkeley, CA; London: University of California Press, 2003), 9. See also Bendelow and Williams, *Transcending the Dualisms*.
20. Bendelow, Gillian A., and Simon J. Williams. "Transcending the Dualisms: Towards a Sociology of Pain". *Sociology of Health & Illness* 17, no. 2 (1995): 139–165.
21. Manderson, Lenore, and Carolyn Smith-Morris. "Introduction: Chronicity and The Experience of Illness". In *Chronic Conditions, Fluid States: Chronicity and the Anthropology of Illness*, edited by Lenore Manderson and Carolyn Smith-Morris (New Brunswick, NJ; London: Rutgers University Press, 2010), 18.
22. A systematic review estimates that the prevalence of chronic pain in the United Kingdom is 43%, affecting 28 million people. See Fayaz, A., P. Croft, R. M. Langford, L. J. Donaldson, and G. T. Jones. "Prevalence of Chronic Pain in the UK: A Systematic Review and Meta-Analysis of Population Studies". *BMJ Open* 6, no. 6 (June 1, 2016). This systematic review of and meta-analysis of population studies includes studies of conditions ranging from Fibromyalgia to chronic neuropathic pain and types of chronic widespread pain. Other studies estimate that 20% of people globally live with pain and that a further 10% is diagnosed with a chronic pain condition each year; see Goldberg, Daniel S., and Summer J. McGee. "Pain as a Global Public Health Priority". *BMC Public Health* 11, no. 1 (2011): 1–5.
23. For example, between financial problems and the intensification of pain, see Rios, R., and A. J. Zautra. "Socioeconomic Disparities in Pain: The Role of Economic Hardship and Daily Financial Worry". *Health Psychol* 30 (2011).
24. Wilkinson, Iain, and Arthur Kleinman. *A Passion for Society: How We Think About Human Suffering*. California Series in Public Anthropology (Oakland, CA: University of California Press, 2016), 95. See also Burgess, Diana J., David B. Nelson, Amy A. Gravely, Matthew J. Bair, Robert D. Kerns, Diana M. Higgins, Michelle van Ryn, Melissa Farmer, and Melissa R. Partin. "Racial Differences in Prescription of Opioid Analgesics for Chronic Noncancer Pain in a National Sample of Veterans". *The Journal of Pain* 15, no. 4: 447–455.
25. Wittgenstein, Ludwig. *Philosophical Investigations* (Oxford: Blackwell, 1958). Wisttgenstein refers to pain in paragraphs 243 to 315.

26. Scarry, Elaine. *The Body in Pain: The Making and Unmaking of the World* (New York; Oxford: Oxford University Press, 1985), 5.
27. Frank, Arthur W. *The Wounded Storyteller: Body, Illness and Ethics* (Chicago; London: University of Chicago Press, 1995), 40.
28. Charon, Rita. "Narrative and Medicine". *New England Journal of Medicine* 350, no. 9 (2004): 862–864; Charon, Rita. *Narrative Medicine: Honoring the Stories of Illness* (New York; Oxford: Oxford University Press, 2006).
29. Jurecic, Ann. *Illness as Narrative* (Pittsburgh: University of Pittsburgh Press, 2012).
30. Jurecic, *Illness as Narrative*, 5.
31. Frank, *The Wounded Storyteller*.
32. Jain, Sarah S. Lochlann. *Malignant: How Cancer Becomes Us* (Berkeley: University of California Press, 2013).
33. Jain, *Malignant*, 66.
34. The cognitive dissonance derived, for Jain, from competing truths held in tandem, holding together 'the factual and the might-well-have-been-or-still-be-otherwise-if-only counterfactual' (Ibid., 4).
35. For example, the assumption that long-term pain naturally leads to disability is at odds with first-person perceptions of pain experience. See Manderson, Lenore, and Carolyn Smith-Morris. "Introduction: Chronicity and the Experience of Illness". In *Chronic Conditions, Fluid States: Chronicity and the Anthropology of Illness*, edited by Lenore Manderson and Carolyn Smith-Morris (New Brunswick, NJ; London: Rutgers University Press, 2010). See also Gonzalez-Polledo, Elena. "Chronic Media Worlds: Social Media and the Problem of Pain Communication on Tumblr". *Social Media + Society* 2, no. 1 (2016): 2056305116628887.
36. Das, *Affliction*.
37. Berlant, Lauren. "Nearly Utopian, Nearly Normal: Post-Fordist Affect in La Promesse and Rosetta". *Public Culture* 19, no. 2 (March 20, 2007): 273–301.
38. Berlant, Lauren. "The Subject of True Feeling: Pain, Privacy and Politics". In *Cultural Pluralism, Identity Politics and the Law*, edited by Austin Sarat and Thomas Kearns (Ann Arbor: The University of Michigan Press, 1999).
39. Berlant, "Nearly Utopian, Nearly Normal," 296. See also Strathern, Marilyn. "The Whole Person and Its Artifacts". *Annual Review of Anthropology* 33, no. 1 (2004): 1–19.

40. Jackson, Jean. ""After a While, No One Believes You": Real and Unreal Pain". In *Pain as Human Experience: An Anthropological Perspective*, edited by Arthur Kleinman, Paul Brodwin, Byron Good, and Mary-Jo DelVecchio Good, 1992; and Jackson, Jean E. *Camp Pain: Talking with Chronic Pain Patients* (Philadelphia, PA: University of Pennsylvania Press, 2000). See also Morris, David B. *The Culture of Pain* (Berkeley: University of California Press, 1991).
41. See Tabor, Abby, Mark J. Catley, Simon Gandevia, Michael A. Thacker, and G. Lorimer Moseley. "Perceptual Bias in Pain: A Switch Looks Closer When It Will Relieve Pain Than When It Won't". *PAIN®* 154, no. 10 (Oct. 2013): 1961–1965. This experimental study, involving 18 naïve individuals, demonstrates that pain is perceived differently according to constantly updated contextual information, but that the environment is differently perceived at different stages of pain onset.
42. Jackson, "After a While, No One Believes You", 140.
43. Ibid., 149.
44. Morris, David B. "Narrative, Ethics and Pain: Thinking with Stories". In *Stories Matter: The Role of Narrative in Medical Ethics*, edited by Rita Charon and Martha Montello (New York; London: Routledge, 2002).
45. Morris, "Narrative, Ethics and Pain," 200.
46. Kleinman et al., *Pain as Human Experience*.
47. Davis, Lennard J. *Enforcing Normalcy: Disability, Deafness, and the Body* (London: Verso, 1995); Ginsburg, Faye, and Rayna Rapp. "Disability Worlds". *Annual Review of Anthropology* 42, no. 1 (2013): 53–68.
48. Goggin, Gerard, and Christopher Newell. *Digital Disability: The Social Construction of Disability in New Media* (Lanham; Oxford: Rowman & Littlefield, 2003); Rice, Carla, Eliza Chandler, Elisabeth Harrison, Kirsty Liddiard, and Manuela Ferrari. "Project Re•Vision: Disability at the Edges of Representation". *Disability & Society* 30, no. 4 (Apr. 21, 2015): 513–527.
49. Carel, Havi, and Ian James Kidd. "Epistemic Injustice in Healthcare: A Philosophial[sic] Analysis". *Medicine, Health Care and Philosophy* 17, no. 4 (Nov. 1, 2014): 529–540. As Carel and Kidd note, a person-centered approach to clinical communication is a core political contention of patient associations in the United Kingdom and North America.
50. Greenhalgh, *Under the Medical Gaze*, 23.
51. Ibid., 206.
52. Morris writes: 'the goal of narrative bioethics is to get the stories into the open, where we can examine their values, sift their conflicts, and explore their power to work on us' Ibid., 213.

53. Carel, Havi. *Illness: The Cry of the Flesh* (Stocksfield: Acumen, 2008), 8.
54. Carel suggests: 'Instead of viewing illness as a local disruption of a particular function, phenomenology turns to the lived experience of this dysfunction. It attends to the global disruption of the habits, capacities and actions of the ill person' Ibid., 8–9.
55. Carel and Kidd, "Epistemic justice and Healthcare".
56. Ibid.
57. Biro, David. *Listening to Pain: Finding Words, Compassion, and Relief* (New York; London: W.W. Norton, 2011), 3.
58. See http://www.iasp-pain.org/Education/Content.aspx?ItemNumber=1519
59. Ihde, Don. *Listening and Voice: Phenomenologies of Sound* (Albany, NY: State University of New York Press, 2007).
60. See Pinch, Trevor, and Karin Bijsterveld. "New Keys to the World of Sound". In *The Oxford Handbook of Sound Studies*, edited by Trevor Pinch and Karin Bijsterveld (Oxford; New York: Oxford University Press, 2012).
61. Ihde, *Listening and Voice*, 200.
62. As do, for instance, sound and words. See Schafer, R. Murray. *The Soundscape: Our Sonic Environment and the Tuning of the World* (Rochester, VT: Destiny Books, 1994). See also Motamedi Fraser, Mariam. *Word: Beyond Language, Beyond Image*. Disruptions. Edited by Paul Bowman (London; New York: Rowman and Littlefield International, 2015).
63. Das, Veena. "Language and the Body: Transactions in the Construction of Pain". In *Social Suffering*, edited by Arthur Kleinman, Veena Das, and Margaret Lock (Berkeley: University of California Press, 1997): 67–92.
64. Das, Veena. *Affliction: Health, Disease, Poverty* (New York: Fordham University Press, 2015).
65. Das, Veena. "Ordinary Ethics". In *A Companion to Moral Anthropology*, edited by Didier Fassin (Oxford: Willey Blackwell, 2012), 133–134.
66. See Manning, Erin. *Relationscapes: Movement, Art, Philosophy*. Technologies of Lived Abstraction (Cambridge, MA: MIT Press, 2009).
67. See Campt, Tina. *Listening to Images* (Durham: Duke University Press, 2017).
68. See Ihde, Don. *Postphenomenology: Essays in the Postmodern Context* (Evanston, IL: Northwestern University Press, 1993); and Ihde, Don. *Postphenomenology and Technoscience: The Peking University Lectures* (Albany, NY: SUNY Press, 2009).

EJ Gonzalez-Polledo is a Lecturer in the Department of Anthropology at Goldsmiths, University of London, with research interests focusing on the anthropology of knowledge: social epistemology, gender, expert models, knowledge transmission, research methods, and data assemblages and infrastructures. EJ is the author of *Transitioning: Matter, Gender, Thought* (Rowman and Littlefield International, 2017) and co-editor of *Queering Knowledge: Analytics, Devices and Investments after Marilyn Strathern* (Routledge, 2018).

2

'The Sad Language of Pain': S. Weir Mitchell, the American Civil War, and Interpreting Physical Suffering

Lucy Bending

> *"If a man positively affirms that he suffers great pain in some portion of his body, it seems to the popular mind absurd for a surgeon to affirm that he does not."*
> Silas Weir Mitchell in Joseph Janvier Woodward (1886)[1]

This chapter's aim is to use the tensions inherent in the claim of J. J. Woodward, the American Civil War Army Assistant Surgeon, as a starting position to consider some of the difficulties in expressing and understanding pain. For Woodward, steeped in the terrible carnage of the Civil War, what constitutes physical pain—what the surgeon envisages as arising from a bodily injury—is at odds with—is perhaps less to be taken into account by the general public than the simple affirmation of that pain by the sufferer. It is only when a patient affirms pain, perhaps performs that pain, that it becomes visible to another. And yet there is, as Woodward is clearly suggesting, a possibility, which flies in the face of popular understanding, that a claim to pain may not be genuine, and may not grow out

---

L. Bending (✉)
University of Reading, Reading, UK

© The Author(s) 2018
EJ Gonzalez-Polledo, J. Tarr (eds.), *Painscapes*,
https://doi.org/10.1057/978-1-349-95272-4_2

of a bodily reality that could be recognized by a medical practitioner. The gap between sufferer and perceiver complicates things, meaning that the experience of pain cannot be simply passed from one person to another, but—if it is not to be seen as 'foreign'—must undergo a process of translation, as words are found, or symptoms are seen and interpreted. The foreignness of pain is not, however, the only difficulty for the surgeon who meets it on the battlefield. Whilst Woodward's fellow Army doctor, renowned neurologist, man of letters, and contemporary, Silas Weir Mitchell, clearly sees pain as a language that is spoken, a language that can articulate suffering, there is another pervasive idea that underlies Mitchell's thought, and it is this that is the focus of this chapter. Pain is not a simple given, but is a kind of performance. Mitchell writes of the 'production of … pain', invoking in that word 'production' both the physical processes of the body in response to trauma and the performance of that pain, that must be staged by sufferers if they are to convince an onlooker of its reality.

This chapter seeks to think about what it means to listen to what Mitchell called 'the sad language of pain', but also what it means to judge the reality of that language against the patient's performance of pain, and how the body reacts rather than what the patient himself says, as the two processes of translation and production run alongside each other, in a negotiation that has implications for the wider understanding of pain and its articulation.

It is by no means new to think about the necessity of listening to those in pain, and, indeed, much of the work done in this area stems from Elaine Scarry's ground-breaking *The Body in Pain* (1985), which articulates both the difficulties of voicing pain and the absolute necessity for hearing, and paying attention to, such voicings of suffering. I am interested here, though, in exploring Weir Mitchell's written responses—predominantly his medical writings, but also, in part, his fiction—to physical suffering, primarily arising from his experience as a Civil War surgeon, and the ways in which he thought about pain and language; of who spoke and who listened, and if, in the end, the evidence offered by the speech of a sufferer was sufficient to necessitate belief in its reality. Mitchell's reputation, as Kay Ferguson Ryals rightly contends, has undergone a profound change since the mid-nineteenth century. He is now predominantly known not for being the foremost American neurologist of the late nineteenth century, repeatedly designated 'the father of American neurology', but as the man who originated the Rest Cure, 'a famous, or infamous, treatment that was widely prescribed to "nervous" American women in the late nineteenth century, and thus as the real-life physician who served as the model for the notorious doctor-husband in Charlotte Perkins-Gilman's "The Yellow Wallpaper", a text which represents the Rest Cure as a devastating form of social control aimed at keeping ambitious women in their "places"'. Ryals is undoubtedly right about this shift in Mitchell's posthumous reputation, and it is a shift that is also recognized in Nancy Cervetti's fascinating exploration of what she sees as the movement in Weir Mitchell from Civil War surgeon, who 'gives voice and visibility to human pain, transcending its mastery of the body and reducing its effect', as the specialist in neurological disorders translates observed bodily experience into a kind of language, to the post-bellum society doctor who 'chooses not to listen' to, refuses fully to see, the 'hysterical' women who come under his care. I think the arc of Cervetti's argument is right, and yet my focus is on the texts written during or immediately after the Civil War: *Gunshot Wounds, and Other Injuries of Nerves* (1864, deemed by Richard Walter, one of Mitchell's biographers, to be 'without a doubt, the most important work published during the Civil War period), in which Mitchell, along with his collaborators George Morehouse and William Keen, voices many of their hesitations over the passage of pain from sufferer to perceiver; 'On Malingering', written with the same two colleagues, which outlines the possibility of duplicity in what people say about their own pain; and *Injuries of Nerves* (1872), a revised and extended rewriting of *Gunshot Wounds*, solely under Mitchell's name, and published seven years after the end of the Civil War. If Cervetti sees a shift from belief to doubt in Mitchell's approach to his patient's painful suffering, then I, whilst concurrently recognizing this movement in his approach to patients, also see his career as riven by doubt, right from the start, at the visible signs of the body, the ways in which these are performed and perhaps manipulated, and how one could understand them. For Mitchell a process is involved in the transmission of pain from one person to another, and it is a process of which Mitchell undoubtedly recognizes the limitations. Whilst, as I will suggest later in this chapter,

Mitchell was determined to professionalize medicine, using as one of the means to this end his insistence on giving the fullest account of what he observed, he nevertheless repeatedly fell back on the recognition that 'we cannot in any way become sure' when looking at another's pain, of what it is, or even if it is real. Absolute knowledge of another's suffering is impossible, though perhaps in that notion of *becoming*, of becoming sure, is an idea of movement towards another, as the patient performs their pain in such a way that it becomes recognizable, and as the watcher responds to that production of pain. The doctor must be convinced by the performance of suffering if he is to believe in its existence.

As Joanna Bourke makes plain in writing about the huge-scale injuries of the Civil War, it brought with it a level of injury that was a huge challenge—and, indeed, an opportunity for the ambitious—for military surgeons. It was, as Bourke argues, 'a conflict of utmost savagery'; a conflict in which over 600,000 American soldiers died, and 30,000 limbs were amputated, a major part of that damage being done by 'the new conical bullet or minié [which] proved to be more damaging to muscle and bone than its predecessors'. Nancy Cervetti extends these claims by writing of the effects of the minié: 'Because the soft lead flattened and broke apart upon hitting the human body, the destruction of tissue, bone, cartilage, and vein was massive. While the entrance wound was the size of a thumb, the exit wound could be the size of a fist, and when hit in the arm or leg, the ball could shatter the bone from a distance of six to ten inches'. Such damage was unprecedented, and demanded new kinds of medical attention, not least because of the damage done to the nerves by the passage of the bullet.

Mitchell recognized the opportunity and, as Richard D. Walter suggests, when, in 1862, his friend and former collaborator the Surgeon General William A. Hammond started to create a hospital designed specifically for soldiers with neurological injuries, Mitchell was determined to be involved, as were his colleagues William Keen and George Morehouse, all three of whom closely collaborated in their medical practice and in the research papers that grew out of this. As Mitchell put it in his autobiographical writings, collected together by Anna Robeson Burr, 'There I began to be interested in cases of nervous disease and wounds of nerves, about which little was then known'. The team of men built up their collection of neurologically wounded soldiers, many of whom were amputees, at the Turner's Lane Hospital in Philadelphia, which came, rather bluntly, to be known as the 'Stump Hospital'. He set up an arrangement whereby he accepted patients that doctors working in other hospitals did not want or know how to treat: he took those with serious neurological damage, and swapped them for more straightforward, commonly encountered patients. As he writes:

> The great bulk of our patients has consisted of men who have been shifted from one hospital to another, and whose cases have been the despair of their surgical attendants. As the wounded of each period of the war have been cured, discharged, invalided, or died, every large hospital had left among the wards two or three or more strange instances of wounds of nerves. Most of these presented phenomena which are rarely seen, and which were naturally foreign to the observation even of those surgeons whose experience was the most extensive and complete.

These 'strange instances', with their unrecognizable pain, are 'foreign' to those who encounter them: they speak a language that cannot be understood, and can only be shifted from one place to another. Indeed, they cannot even be properly seen:

> Nowhere were these cases described at length in the text-books, and, except in a single untranslated French book, their treatment was passed over in silence; while even in the volume in question but a limited class of nerve lesions was discussed. In the great monographs on military surgery, this defect is still so complete, that wounds of nerves are there related rather as curiosities and as matters for despair than with any view to their full clinical study and systematic treatment.

If Elaine Scarry argues that pain is wrapped in silence because it cannot be articulated, then the silence here is different: it is the silence of the medical practitioners, baffled by the severity of the injuries they encountered, who chose not to confront the phenomenon of pain. Silence grows from the unwillingness to describe symptoms and find treatments, rather than from the failure of the doctor to recognize the words of the wounded soldier. Mitchell in his Civil War medical textbooks recognizes and seeks to redress this 'defect'.

It is the reason—and Mitchell's explanation—for this lack of knowledge about injured soldiers with neurological damage that interests me in this chapter, as it points not just towards the unusualness of such wounds, and their concurrent pain, but also both a refusal to listen to such suffering, a refusal to engage with its strangeness, and that strangeness itself which made it seem that the body of the neurologically wounded soldier was speaking a language that could not be understood. If pain could only be either a 'curiosity' or a matter for despair, then the patients in pain could not be easily engaged with. The refusal to engage turns the pain into something else, something beyond medical reach, making it an object of fear.

This doubt as to what pain is, and whether it can be recognized, crosses over into the article, 'On Malingering, Especially in Regard to Simulation of Diseases of the Nervous System', which fascinatingly grapples with the question of how to tell if disease is real or feigned. The article, stemming from close engagement with soldiers suffering from neurological disorders, has at its centre the difficulty of knowing for certain if someone else's bodily suffering is real. All kinds of disorder and disease were feigned by soldiers seeking discharge from the Army, from deafness, to diarrhoea, to paralysis, but as the three authors recognized, there is something particular about pain and its invisibility, its reliance on verbal testimony that made it a unique symptom. As Mitchell writes, while 'pain is not a feigned disease, [it is] the most easily feigned symptom, the most difficult and often most apparently cruel to gainsay or deny, and, at the same time, the most available stronghold to which the malingerer can resort'. Doubting pain is—as we saw Woodward assert—in itself a kind of cruelty, and, indeed, this cruelty could stretch to strikingly harsh treatment at the hands of medical practitioners who refused to believe in the reality of the supposed malingerer's pain. Mitchell cites the case of an English naval surgeon who 'compelled a suspected malingerer, even by flogging, to lift and swing an eighteen pound weight with his arms, despite the most earnest entreaties and asseverations of agonizing pain in his shoulder'. Only after his 'earnest entreaties' have been denied, was the surgeon called on to evacuate 'two pounds of purulent matter' from the shoulder. The evacuated pus spoke louder than the man's words, which were insufficient to bear effective testimony to his suffering. In Mitchell's eyes, the surgeon becomes 'the author of this cruelty', as his doubt, and the flogging that follows from it, is a more coherent and powerful narrative than the sailor's own words.

Mitchell's doubts over the nature and action of power and the validity of speech in the face of pain come to the fore in his contention that it is difficult to court-martial a malingerer, 'since in many a case in which it is morally certain that the man is a malingerer, it is yet impossible to swear to it'. Medical certainty falls at the hurdle of 'such evidence as will convince a court of non-professional men'. Bodily suffering, or the lack of it, is turned into 'evidence', and, in this process, becomes a form of argument rather than a somatic reality. If the soldier can put forward convincing evidence of his pain, then the layman will not doubt it. As Mitchell counters, the malingerer 'frequently tells a pitiful story', or will 'whimper and even sob in an unmanly manner, which in itself alone should produce suspicion'. Such unmanly sobbing—what looks to the layman like the proof of pain—becomes in the eyes of the surgeon evidence of his duplicity. 'No men are so apt to exaggerate and overact their part, nor any so apt to endeavour to move belief by backing their assertions by repetition and affirmation, as those who feign simple pain. Such means are necessary to bolster doubtful assertion only'. Pain is a performance, and yet it is one that can be shamelessly overacted. And yet there is another possibility, as Mitchell recognizes that the surgeon, faced with an enactment of pain, can become *too* convinced by his own evidence, too impressed by his 'dexterity in detecting deception', and gets to the point where 'in every "back case" we shall see a malingerer'. No performance can be sufficient to persuade, as every soldier falls under suspicion. What matters to him here is what is *seen*, rather than what is *heard*: the doctor's power to observe is more significant than the patient's power to assert his suffering. What one expects, what one is paid to detect, stands in the way of clear vision, of the ability to listen to the 'most earnest entreaties and asseverations', until one sees only deceit.

Mitchell's article shores itself up with technologies and practices that will disclose deceit, that will be able to discern the difference between real pain and faked pain, that will see through the duplicitous claims and overacted miseries of the malingerer to the real bodily pain of the genuinely suffering—the galvanism that will jerk the malingerer's muscles into action, the ether that will take away the body's ability to control its actions, the spies who will watch the doubted soldier while he thinks no one is looking, the detailed observation of the way in which the supposedly lame man uses a walking stick. It becomes a battle between doctor and soldier as to whose words are to be the more powerful, as the soldier sees pain as 'the most available stronghold' available to him, a fortress that cannot be breached, whilst the surgeon counters with the anaesthesia that will dupe the doubted man's body into betraying itself, and which is 'summoned as a reserve to decide the fortunes of a doubtful day'. The body's response—when decoupled from the conscious will by ether—is more compelling, more truthful, than the man's spoken words. Diagnosis is a battlefield. There can be no absolute certainty, but the strongest argument will prevail. And yet, in the face of this, 'such cases' as that of the flogged English sailor with the agonizingly purulent arm 'have', as Mitchell puts it, 'made us wary' in this battle between doubt and certainty. As he goes on to suggest, 'It is unfortunately the fact, that one rogue throws a shadow of suspicion on a dozen honest men', and it is for this reason that Mitchell deliberately chooses to 'name' these wrongly doubted soldiers, or at least draw attention to their existence in 'On Malingering'. In writing this treatise on malingerers, caught between compassion and caution, Mitchell both exerts his power as one who can determine the fate of the wounded, and voices his own doubt, and speaks the real pain of soldiers out loud and, in so doing, acknowledges the reality of their suffering. The danger is, as he all too sharply recognizes, that 'in endeavouring to do justice to the government, we be led unwittingly, to do injustice to the man'.

And yet Union surgeons have a duty to the government they serve: malingerers must be found out and sent back to the field of battle. In fighting mode, Mitchell makes plain that 'where no other evidence than the man's assertion of pain exist, he should be sent back to his regiment' to fight. Assertion of pain is insufficient and fakeable, and yet the caveat that Mitchell adds to this statement is at the heart of the matter: 'But it should be understood that "no other evidence" is to be accurately determined'. Such a decision must not be based on a whim, but on proper, extensively documented, medical grounds. *Gunshot Wounds* insists on the seeking of evidence, on just such accurate determination of symptoms:

Our materials for this study consist of about one hundred and twenty cases, all of which have been carefully reported in our note books during the past year. No labor [sic] has been spared in making these clinical histories as perfect and full as possible. Those only who have devoted themselves to similar studies will be able to appreciate the amount of time and care which have been thus expended. We indulge the hope that we shall leave on record a very faithful clinical study of nerve injuries, and that we shall have done something at least toward lessening the inevitable calamities of warfare.

'Full' description on the doctors' part will somehow make up for the inability to trust or to understand the 'foreignness' of the patients' language. Mitchell's framing comments here clearly establish the qualities that he values and the difficulties faced. All of the texts written during the Civil War by the doctors at the Stump Hospital relied on shared information, as the three doctors who worked together decided who would write up which of the clinical observations that they made for publication. There is an insistence on information being unmediated; it must come straight from notes taken at the time of medical examination. No artefacts will be introduced by the passage of time nor by the processes of memory and forgetfulness. Mitchell's stress is on the absolute care of the note takers: conditions are 'carefully reported', they are 'as perfect and full as possible', they have had great 'time and care … expended' on them, and they are 'a very faithful clinical study'. The stress is very clearly on a direct transcription of the medical case itself. Ernest Earnest recounts the meticulous attention to detail of the record keeping at the Stump Hospital, making plain that 'a single case may take up five to nine pages of foolscap'. Conventions for case notes were standardized to ensure the 'full' account that Mitchell required, and cases could be followed for up to two years in these notes. As Kay Ferguson Ryals compellingly argues in her dissertation, *Bedside Manners and the Social Body: S. Weir Mitchell and the Virtues of Medical Practice*, 'Mitchell's team' at the Stump Hospital went beyond well-kept case notes, and 'pioneered novel methods of clinical research, including innovative principles of hospital management and record-keeping'. The connection is not made explicit, but Ryals moves on to discuss the state of the American medical profession during and after the American

Civil War, drawing into prominence the fact that 'the 1830s and 40s saw the end of most attempts at state regulation and licensing of physicians', which left the field open to an unregulated and poorly trained medical profession. If one counter move to this was the formation of the American Medical Association in 1847, it seems evident that Mitchell and his colleagues' meticulous attention to detail—to close observation and accurate record keeping—was a different kind of reaction to this, one also born from what Stephanie Browner, writing of the 1850s, sees as the contest between 'earlier universalist therapeutics', that saw all illness as arising from the same cause, and its companion, taking shape in 'contemporary populist practitioners like Samuel Thomson who claimed that most patients and most illness could be treated by one regimen or a single tonic'. Mitchell's insistence on keeping meticulous note of individual circumstances and symptoms cuts against this universalist thrust. For Mitchell and his colleagues it was only through close observation of the individual case and its particularities, and the tracing of its path through accurate record keeping, that effective medical advance and cure could come.

Mitchell knew, however, as did his colleagues, that this 'very faithful clinical study' was beset with difficulty and error. Human error came into play as Morehouse delayed his writing up of the collected notes on epilepsy for so long that they were destroyed in a fire in his study, and could never—much to Mitchell's distress, and presumably annoyance—be published. More significant, however, than this human tardiness, was the nature of the conditions studied, and the pain encountered and endured by the soldiers in the wards. Notes could be taken, and yet pain remained elusive, tricky, deceptive; it is this trickery, intentional or otherwise on the part of the patient that led to the article on malingering.

Not only could pain be misleading, but the nature of medical practice—its necessary extension over time—could also lead to misunderstanding. Mitchell's awareness of the difficulties of recapitulating experience, particularly as it takes shape in the gap between the time of writing and the time of encounter with the patient in pain, and the possibility of forgetfulness and the inaccuracies of mental and spatial distance from the patient, really comes to the fore in the later text, *Injuries of Nerves*, which looks back and works through case histories recorded during the Civil War. In this retrospective account of his time at the

Stump Hospital, he assuages his doubts over the veracity of his writing by claiming 'In delineating this form of pain'—and here he is writing of causalgia—the disease that is now particularly associated with Weir Mitchell—'perhaps I cannot do better than transfer to these pages the account originally written whilst I was seeing almost daily numbers of persons suffering as I have described them'. It is a claim fraught with, if not contradictions, at least tensions. The 'delineation' of which he writes suggests a kind of clinical accuracy, but also provides only an outline, leaving a space within the medical terminology to be filled in by the patient's own experience, or, indeed, by artefacts stemming from the passage of time. This is not the only moment of hesitation in a claim that ends in confidence. Tentativeness suffuses the negative formulation of 'perhaps I cannot do better ...' and results in a desire simply to 'transfer' experience from the earlier notebooks to the later textbook in a process that avoids the contamination of time, and perhaps undue reflection. Mitchell recognizes early on in the text that the interval between experience and the writing of that experience has its advantages, in making it possible 'to collect ... such details of later history as were needed to clear up or complete the story of symptoms or prognosis'—at the moment of pain the story is incomplete, and perhaps the physician responds inadequately or simply cannot see something that will only appear in the fullness of time. And yet, after this moment of recognition that what one sees might not be the whole picture, comes the assertion of the doctor's authority. The closing phrase, insisting that the patients suffered 'as I described them', shifts the balance—and it is the doctor who holds the template, and the sufferer who fits himself to it. Description and experience here are identical—though the reverberating doubts of the earlier part of the sentence cannot surely disappear into thin air.

There are other difficulties, of course, in Mitchell's descriptions of physical suffering. The doubt is not just that things will change over time, but that the information gathered by the doctor is somehow questionable. Mitchell repeatedly falls back on such phrases as 'the pain which they described', allowing in that the possibility that the soldier in pain, even if he is not a malingerer deliberately endeavouring to deceive, is not correct in his representation of what he feels. In his account of the sensations of men who have been shot, Mitchell points out that

Of them by far the larger number felt, when shot, as though someone had struck them sharply with a stick, and one or two were so possessed with this idea at the time, that they turned to accuse a comrade of the act, and were unpleasantly surprised to discover, from the flow of blood, that they had been wounded.

Pain, coming out of the blue, creates an idea that possesses the mind and takes over, creating a story that makes sense of what has happened, and which cannot easily be displaced. 'The pain which they described', as Mitchell well knows, is subject to this creative impulse, as pain creates stories. It is this impulse to make sense of a painful sensation that causes further difficulties of belief. Mitchell goes further than suggesting a gap between the experience and the word used to catch it, in suggesting that the patient, suffering from causalgia, outlines 'a state of torture, which can hardly be credited' and behaves 'with a care which seems absurd'. Both of these terms veer between acceptance of what is conveyed by the patient and a sense that the patient's behaviour has gone beyond the credible. As Mitchell goes on to write of one such patient in *Injuries of Nerves*, 'At last the patient grows hysterical, if we may use the only term which describes the facts'. It is an interesting phrase. There is a word that accurately describes what the doctor observes, and yet it is a word associated with women rather than with injured soldiers. Mitchell's hesitation over using the description 'hysteria' is one that is bound up in decorum and gender politics—the question is 'may he' use the word hysterical in relation to soldiers; is it permissible to do so? In writing of the same patient, a man called H. in those notes, age 39, and designated Case 33, we are told that 'my notes describe him on entering our wards as presenting the following symptoms', and what follows is the quotation of Mitchell's own notes, made at the time: there is a deliberate choice to leave the language as it originally was, a choice not to edit or to remove ambivalence. The case notes read:

> The hyperaesthesia of the palm was excessive, so that even to blow on it seemed to give pain. He kept it wrapped up and wet ... After a few weeks of this torment he became so sensitive that the rustle of a paper or of a woman's dress, the sound of feet, ... all appeared to increase his pain. His countenance at this time was worn, pinched, anaemic, his temper irritable, and his manner so odd that some of the attendants believed him insane.

When questioned as to his condition he assured me that every strong moral emotion made him worse, - anger or disappointment expressing themselves cruelly in the aching limb.

It is a fascinating account, because the language of the piece is pulled in so many different directions. The passage is full of the phrases Mitchell came to rely on—'it seemed' and 'it appeared'—and we hear the voice of the sceptical medical practitioner, made all the more present by the acceptance of this earlier version of events as it is re-read and published in 1872. But we also hear, I think, buried in Mitchell's account, the desperation of the soldier who felt the need to *'assure'* Mitchell that strong emotion made things worse for his pain. The soldier goes beyond telling how things are; his words fail to find acceptance and he must push into persuasion. In these surroundings where the patient is not necessarily to be believed, and the attendants may have ways of understanding entirely at odds with the doctor and with the patient, the pain itself becomes an actor in this exchange. H.'s emotions must have a voice, and as such, as Mitchell puts it, they 'express themselves—they find their own kind of language—cruelly in the aching limb'. That they express themselves 'cruelly' suggests a kind of personality to pain: they do not simply press out meaning, but do it with a kind of malice. Such delineations clearly link Mitchell's embodiments of pain back to such pictures as James Gillray's 1799 cartoon, 'The Gout', in which the inflamed foot of a man suffering from gout, is fiercely attacked by an evil-looking, sharp-talented devil, intent on sinking claws and teeth into the tender foot.

This version of pain—one buzzing with the idea that pain can take on an embodied form, can have a mind and behaviour of its own that is somehow outside the remit of the body—at times infuses Mitchell's medical writing. Writing of organs that perhaps only once in a lifetime feel pain, he asks if it is possible that there should be a system of nerves dedicated only to pain that may never, or only ever rarely, be called upon:

> Are we to suppose that there exist always in these organs pain nerves, and that only once, perhaps, in a lifetime these filaments are to be aroused into activity? Or, as regards the skin, how shall we deal with the like difficulty if we choose to believe that everywhere are peculiar nerve fibres devoted only to transmitting painful sensations?

Mitchell does not have the answer to this question of whether there are specific pain pathways, but his descriptions of the actions of the nerves carrying pain—their arousal and their devotion—suggests something living; something outside the realms of the purely neurological. Alongside this, for the physician, it is a matter of *choosing* to believe if there are dedicated nerves for pain. It is as though two worlds are colliding: the world of observation, knowledge, and note-taking, and an older world view that relies on belief and a sense of the embodiment of pain in a malign shape. It is no mistake that when Mitchell gives his opinion on dedicated nerve pathways, he puts it in terms of his willingness to accept his conclusions: 'I am unwilling', he says, 'in view of the facts, to look upon pain as a distinct sense with afferent tracks peculiar to itself'.

The doctor, uncertain of the functioning of the nervous system, recognizes that his observations alone are insufficient: his judgement relies on his willingness to perceive things in a particular way; his willingness to translate the foreignness of the body into terms that he can understand. Pain, as Mitchell insists throughout his writing, speaks a foreign language. In trying to understand he writes of the possibility of a system of nerves devoted specifically to pain, and distinct from the system concerned with heat or touch: 'it is', he writes, 'as if through a single tube were spoken various languages which could be only understood when, at its farther end, they reached the ear of the hearer native to each form of speech'. All kinds of impulses—sensation and pain—travel along the same nerves, like a message through a speaking tube, and it is only when they reach the end point that they are interpreted. The listener dedicated to warmth interprets the sensation in that way, whilst the listener listening out for pain will hear that as it comes thundering through the speaking tube. Mechanical disturbances along the path of the nerve are felt as pain, as the nerve translates the sensation into what Mitchell calls 'this sad language'. Pain, as Mitchell found from his experience with malingerers, could be—and, indeed, was—faked for the patient's advantage, and yet the difficulty lay in not allowing the knowledge of this to preclude the possibility of its real existence. This analogy of speaking tube and nervous system gives a way of understanding Mitchell's own response to the pain of his patients, and their desire and difficulty in communicating it. It was the purpose of the doctor to place himself at the end of the speaking tube, and not just to hear, but to interpret, the language that came to his ear, in ways that others—even those in the same physical position—were unable to do without such training and experience. The shot man, who interpreted his gunshot wound as a blow from a stick, equally had his ear to the end of the speaking tube, and yet was profoundly mistaken in his interpretation of his pain. Mitchell's ability to hear correctly, medically, grows from the experience, note-keeping, and training unavailable to the individual soldier trying to make sense of his experience.

This difficulty of interpretation, of making sense of the pain of another, comes to the fore in Mitchell's extraordinary short story, 'The Case of George Dedlow', originally published in 1866 in The *Atlantic Monthly*, a non-medical journal, whose subtitle named it 'a magazine of literature, art, and politics'. In it, George Dedlow, a Union lieutenant, is repeatedly wounded whilst fighting in the Civil War, and finds himself, by the end of the story, in the Stump Hospital, having had all of his limbs amputated, until he is no more than 'a useless torso, more like some strange larval creature than anything of human shape'. Mitchell published the story anonymously, and its first-person account of Dedlow's distress and pain caused a huge response among its readership, who, despite its ludicrousness—Dedlow gets in touch with his lost legs in a seance at the end of the story, which, because they have been stored in alcohol, stagger around drunkenly—believed it to be a true account. As D. G. Kline argues, the story became 'immensely popular. Many readers felt that it was fact … They sent mail to this fictional person, attempted to visit him at the hospital, and even raised money for him and left it at the hospital'. Mitchell's intention was not to deceive, and, indeed, as he wrote after the republication of the text in 1900, he 'certainly could never have conceived it possible that his humorous sketch …., and especially its absurd ending, would for a moment mislead anyone'. The comedy of Mitchell's story got lost somewhere in translation, and in a way that embodies the power of pain, both to create stories and to shift between origin and hearer, a nation traumatized by recent war failed to see the absurdity that Mitchell thought was all too evident, but could only hear only the 'sad language of pain'. As Joanna Bourke astutely puts it, 'Dedlow's fate was unusual, but imaginable to readers still reeling from the carnage of the war'. This makes it all too plain that pain cannot exist in a vacuum; that it is always subject to the imagination both of the self, who tries to make sense of an absolutely strange sensation, and to others who find themselves in relation to it. In a strange twist, Mitchell found himself incensed when, 30 years after the end of the Civil War, he found that his careful record keeping and writing up of his notes—the keystone of his professionalism and accuracy—was doubted by 'an English writer [who] declares that he has never seen causalgia such as we saw it from 1861 to 1864', and therefore doubted the validity of Mitchell's claims. Mitchell responds by writing of 'men worn out with marching, soaked with malaria, and exhausted by exposure and diarrhoea, [and subjects] of wounds from mini-balls', and yet, as Mitchell himself was apt to do, the English critic was willing to rely only on what he had seen, rather than what had heard from another. As Richard Walter points out, 'in spite of the bolstering evidence … the "burning pain" syndrome [causalgia] seemed too bizarre, too far removed from common medical experience to be completely accepted'. The untrustworthiness of the patient transferred itself to the doctor, as Mitchell's own engagement with pain came under suspicion.

Note

1. Woodward, Joseph Janvier. *Outline of the Chief Camp Diseases of the United States Armies as Observed During the Present War. A practical Contribution to Military Medicine* (Philadelphia: Lippincott, 1886), 326.

Lucy Bending is a Lecturer in English at the University of Reading. Her first book, *The Representation of Bodily Pain in Late Nineteenth-Century English Culture*, explores the way understandings of pain are shaped by their cultural context. Her work has continued to engage with the ways in which writers try to find language for elusive bodily experiences.

3

An Essay on the Space Outside Pain Where the Poem Takes Place

Jude Rosen

In the Beginning … The Pain That Gave Birth to Words

Acquiring a condition that wouldn't go away, I acquired new words: sigmoidoscopy, endoscopy, enteroclysis, new distinctions and nuances of language: barium meal, barium enema, barium follow-through. The earliest incident of my 'disease career' that I recall relates to my encounter with a sigmoidoscopy, lying on my front, with my lower half uncovered. A man came into the room whom I had never met, who did not address me. He held out his pudgy pink fingers and the nurse stuffed them into creamy plastic gloves like pork sausages into skins. He then delved into my back passage with long silver instruments—Roald Dahl caricatures of giant scissors and pincers on stilts—and left, and I never saw him again. Not a word was exchanged with me. I was diagnosed, without any follow-up consultation, with irritable bowel syndrome and sent to a psychiatrist—a common treatment at the time for women who had

J. Rosen (✉)
London, UK

Crohn's disease but not men similarly misdiagnosed—that ensured I was not treated for Crohn's disease for another four years.

I wrote a ditty:

> Dr. Dick, Dr. Dick
> you silly old prick,
> your brain is soft
> and your skin is thick.

I hesitate to call it a poem as it imitated a nursery rhyme, written out of revenge for the physical humiliation and denial of me as a sentient being with feelings—and also of the reality of my illness and pain as a woman.

The writing itself also embodies my subordination to the doctor in the clinic, because it reproduces the infantile position in which he put me. The reason why this incident was seminal for my writing on pain was because I was belittled as though I were a child, and the ditty is the infantile response of cat-calling, sexual insult, contempt for the intelligence of the person—all the ways children in the playground hit back at their elders and 'betters' when they feel put down and powerless.

The poems that followed were not driven by revenge, but by the will to resist, refusing to be confined and defined solely by pain, by building alliances with the world outside chronic pain, of countering its dominance and power through connecting with others and—notionally at least—with a wider public of readers.

Of course this was not a wholly conscious strategy, but one which evolved. Nor was it explicitly political, as resistance in writing takes place, first of all, in and through language—itself a social, cultural and cognitive structure. It was at first a response to make sense of what had happened to me, to get through, to survive. But a consciousness grew with the experience of pain and writing about it which had political implications and, potentially at least, effects. By writing poetry out of pain, I wanted to challenge the representation of pain in our culture as the outcome of individual physical or psychic weakness or moral failure, and reframe the understanding of pain through empathy. Such empathy, as I have experienced it, affords the writer respite from suffering and transforms the relationship to the other—the reader—enabling the sufferer to come out of silent isolation and connect to the wider culture. And while chronic pain ravages the body and self, writing is an act of creation that leaves something irrevocable behind which has a life of its own.

Pain, Memory and Empathy

In seeking to create a connection with readers, audience, public, the universal aspect of pain offers a common starting point. As Susan Sontag points out

> Everyone who is born holds dual citizenship in the kingdom of the well and the kingdom of the sick. Although we all prefer to use only the good passport, sooner or later each of us is obliged, at least for a spell, to identify ourselves as citizens of that other place.[1]

Outside of the traumas of war and torture, we have all experienced pain of some kind, through the trials of birth and the first few weeks of life, childhood diseases, injuries, adult illnesses and accidents, psychic pain and distress, whether or not these have been compounded by the very unequal ordeals of poverty, social violence, the absence of effective health and welfare services. Usually these experiences are not as severe, persistent or corrosive as chronic pain, but they are a point of commonality and connection across cultures and social divisions. Persistent pain is not incommensurable, or beyond the comprehension of those who are free of its ardent pursuit.

A starting point for fostering empathy is to rekindle their own memory of moments of physical and psychic pain to enable a connection with the suffering of those who endure it chronically, for whom it is an integral and inescapable part of everyday life. Also to invoke and critically draw on the language of the culture through which pain has been framed, represented and understood. And further, to find metaphors which connect to universal or widespread experiences which can be associated with the demands and effects of chronic pain, even if the reader has not experienced it her- or himself.

However, this bridge to the reader encounters a number of obstacles—apart from the limited reach and reception of the written word, especially poetry.

In 'Pain has an Element of Blank', Emily Dickinson identifies the totalitarian utterness of pain—beginning and ending the poem with the word 'Pain', capital P: Pain—has an Element of Blank/It cannot recollect/When it begun—or if there were/A time when it was not'.[2] The poem repeatedly underlines pain's relationship to time and memory as negative: 'cannot', 'was not', 'It has no Future'; its lines are short and broken and at the end of the poem the past is swallowed up between the 'Infinite' and more of ever-recurring 'New Periods – of Pain'. As in life, so in the poem, pain has taken over everything and devoured time, leaving no contrast or difference, no change or diminishing of its power.

This all-embracing character of chronic pain is not only overwhelming for the sufferer but can also feel overwhelming and frightening for the reader and breed aversion to dwelling on it. Even where the poem has found the language, form and music that resonate with readers or audience, it will come up against resistance to confronting such pain. In the spell when pain overpowers, it tends to induce forgetfulness, blanking out personal memory as Emily Dickinson epitomised in another short lyric: 'There is a pain—so utter/It swallows substance up—/Then covers the Abyss with Trance—/So Memory can step/Around—across—upon it—.'[3]

A sense of wellbeing tends towards a blithe unawareness of the sensory, neurological and physiological processes of the body, its demands and limits: through youthful abandon—to drink, drugs, reckless sports, the belief nothing can happen to you, mothers' hazy recall of labour pains and childbirth .... Even when tell-tale signs of illness or disease become evident, often they are consciously overridden. This lack of awareness of the corrosive effects of long-term pain hardens into institutional insensitivity and indifference despite discrimination against the disabled being officially outlawed. Chronic illness where there are persistent relapses or long periods of absence, without cover available, is a grey area where the chronically sick can be seen as a nuisance, incapable of doing the job or as unreliable. Institutions driven primarily by utilitarian imperatives mechanically apply the short-term expectations of recovery from temporary conditions to chronic illness, demanding, 'When are you returning to work?'

The same kind of question operates under the prevailing neo-liberal, cost-cutting residual welfare regime. Official public discourse displays punitive suspicion of sufferers of persistent disease and pain as work-shy dependents. Welfare need has been recast according to the Victorian distinction between the deserving and undeserving poor, with cruel, even lethal consequences for people with long-term illness or disablement as the Ken Loach film *I, Daniel Blake* painfully highlights. Between December 2011 and February 2014, 2380 people died within two weeks of being declared 'fit for work' and having their benefit entitlement (Employment and Support Allowance) removed.[4]

So building empathy against the fear of being overwhelmed by pain and the weight of necessary forgetting, with which most healthy people unconsciously protect themselves, calls for the special persuasive power of art—its capacity to surmount barriers and defences, override resistance, think critically, see things from a different angle, satirise. In this way it can transcend differences and reach shared emotions and acknowledgement of common human frailties and capacities of resilience.

Writing can enable a point of contact with the other, whether reading public or live audience, who do not experience chronic pain … by making a connection with the pain they have experienced and the language in which pain is represented and framed in the culture which we collectively inhabit.

In this, writing suffers far less from the numbing effect of visual media exposé to horror and atrocity. In *Regarding the Pain of Others*, Sontag highlights the difference in the *Paris Match* advertising slogan of 1949 between 'the weight of words, the shock of photos'[5] to underline the immediacy of visual impact. But chronic pain cannot be conveyed by shock, rather by gradual build-up, implacable persistence, draining relentlessness, which photography as a medium is not well suited to convey. Chronic pain works monotonously by repetition, cumulatively by accretion; even when acute periods are replaced by stable periods, relapses occur …. Like music, poetry deals in repetition and variations: in rhymes, echoes, assonance, alliteration; chorus, refrain and forms such as the villanelle, pantoum and sestina—with patterns of repeating lines. By use of repetition, poetry can enact memory but in each repetition the setting has changed and the momentum is different, so each memory recalling the previous sound of a word, phrase or line is also different in the context of the whole, the tone and meaning shift as the poem moves on. Yet it is hard to find a body of work which has imaginatively addressed chronic pain in poetry … unlike the ubiquitous poems of doomed love which explore the broken heart!

Transforming Pain Through Writing

Pain is a totalising subject that takes over the living self and turns it into an object, a slave to its dictates, demeaning and often infantilising, reducing you to base physical functions and processes, so you lose language and voice, the sense of your self and shape of your life.

Through writing, the self aspires to, and at least temporarily attains, a place outside of pain to investigate it, so a reversal takes place in which pain becomes the object and in the process, the author becomes the subject who defines it. To resist being subsumed by pain requires a space outside of it, maybe only a crack from which to write:

> **Reflection**[6]
>
> Caught in the mirror in a casual glance
> startled eyes against the bleached walls stare back
> from the sylph face of a girl without substance.
> I glimpse another being in her lack
> of form and flesh and in her etherealness
> in the shower room with a single shower head,
> see the dead awakening. Then as I dress,
> the autumn skirt falls off like slough I've shed.
> I see myself slipping through a hairbreadth's crack
> into limbo, from where I wonder how
> to reconstitute life's tissue and come back,
> but wondering transports me to here and now.
> Though substance has vanished in thin air…
> mind absorbs the matter and stops me going spare.

3 An Essay on the Space Outside Pain Where the Poem Takes Place

In making pain an object to be explored imaginatively, represented and communicated, the suffering self is transformed to some degree so that the hold pain exerts is circumvented. The subject and object change in the poem—from the alienated girl without substance, who is not at first recognised, to the 'I' who catches sight of her in the mirror and holds onto her even through the fears of disappearing and dying. By becoming the subject, however tenuously, through self-reflexive thinking, the poem enacts the failure of pain to close off the mind, stops it whittling away at her substance and sanity.

In 'Crohn heroine' the distancing from the pain takes place through a drug-induced hallucination in hospital which enables the sufferer to see the damage of the disease—the rusted chassis of her body from the outside, up in the air looking down, and experience respite from pain as far away, on the end of a telephone line, albeit still connected:

Crohn heroine[7]

The bed had a ramp, a 'sit up and take notice of you' bed with a plastic undersheet to catch any slip ups. The sheets were creased, with brownish streaks, dried blood—they weren't for changing. The bed leaked fluids it didn't have. In the middle of the night I sat bolt upright and naked *Are there mosquitoes here?* I inquired. *What do you think you're at the seaside?* the nurse retorted.

> The itching went on all night and then at six everyone
> woke up when I conked out. My bed floated in the sea, the pain
> was on the end of a telephone line I could hear faintly
> in the distance. The bed blew up into a lilo that floated
> into the Mediterranean—middle earth between
> the ephemeral and the divine—and I dived under water
> exploring corals and angel fish. Seaweed garlanded
> my arms, tangling with the telephone wires—I wasn't completely
> cut off… I floated out of my body looking down
> from the sea clouds on the husk with its dented
> metal casing and crumpled mesh. Sparklers were shooting out,
> fizzing and spurting. I heard inchoate shouting far away.
> After *Give me high five*, I rejoined the lilo that blew up
> into an airship and I was tripping on the bed in an air bubble.

At first it hit me as a vacuum—the sticky electricity stopped
crackling in my head and my blood tamed and then
I felt heat, real heat that claws black to ash, cools lava
to pumice stone, lolling froth and burning and I knew
there must be air though there was nothing to breathe
but hot froth, stained sheets with frothing magma surging up,
retching up from the earth's bowels, where mud
settles, charcoal sediments. It left fossils in the mould
like crows' feet in bark and whitened bone of empty sockets.

First in prose and then in a dreamlike sequence that mutates into long, gushing lines, full of heightened sensations and hyperactivity of clashing metals and minerals, tangled wires, crackling electricity, volcanic explosion, the poem enacts the pain and violence of the disease itself—the damage it wrought, laying waste the body and sucking the marrow out of the narrator, reducing her to bone. Here the 'heroine' of the title plays out ironically in more than one way.

The act of communicating pain through writing, or other art forms, can be an act taking power back and away from pain, a triumph over its omnipotence, by defining and understanding it; by the aesthetic satisfaction of having created an imaginative work that is independent of its ravages and even of the sufferer who gave birth to it; by the connection, both cognitive and social, between the sufferer/artist and public. By breaking the silence, the writer comes out of the isolation that pain inflicts. This also entails redefining the self, not primarily by the chronic pain suffered and illness endured and lived with, but by the acts of witness or resistance, the relationships built in spite of it and the work created which lives in defiance of it.

While reclaiming subjectivity is an essential and powerful step to recovering some control over your life, at the same time it does not necessarily further the development of your writing, if being 'a chronic pain sufferer' becomes the badge of artistic identity. It is a paradox that you can only achieve art by diminishing ego, trying to curb or even dissolve its obtruding shadow, as poetry rarely works well as a vehicle of confessional 'self-expression' or obsessive spillage of secrets. The experience of pain, as of any other subject matter, has to be transformed through the art form—in poetry through language, linguistic form and play—to set it free. To be a poet who suffers from chronic pain means being free to write any kind of poem on any subject, not being confined to a label of 'poet of chronic pain'.

Pain and Intentionality

This relationship between pain and writing bears a particular resemblance to Elaine Scarry's theorisation of pain and imagination as being at opposite ends of a continuum including all sensory perception.[8] Whereas the imagination is *only* knowable through the external symbolic objects it creates in the real world, pain is seen as at the opposite pole having no material referents and objects outside itself, no feeling for anything other than itself, no capacity for outward representation.

The senses operate close to the pole of the imagination in conveying external objects (you see the picture through your eyes; feel the wind and sun on your skin; hear music and different voices with your ears) but if the sensations become too strong to the point of discomfort or harm, the focus shifts from the objects sensed to the sensory process itself and to the part of the body which is hurting. Arriving close to the pole of pain, sensory overload or damage precludes taking in objects as consciousness becomes focused on the internal sensory process itself.

One of the crucial insights of her work is that pain is an entirely interior experience without external referents or material form. Yet this does not mean that pain is inexpressible in language, although it makes it harder to communicate as it eats away at the means to make it known— at the energy, capacity for thought and creative powers of the chronic sufferer. Scarry's theorisation is rather too emphatic and totalising, because the intensity of pain is not constant, but can vary with periods of lower intensity, be dulled or even relieved for periods of time, just as the senses still operate to some degree conveying objects even when there is some discomfort or pain from using them. Chronic pain is not usually continuous—unbroken and uniform—but tends to be continual over years, episodic and indeterminate, without it having an end, or the sufferer knowing if or when it will end. Chronic pain sufferers have to find the physical and mental resources to write and the language, metaphors and music … and silence with which to tackle pain.

Scarry defines the imagination, in contrast to pain, as an intentional object without an intentional state—that is creating imaginative objects—artworks or new ideas—without self-reflexive awareness of the creative process. Physical pain, on the contrary, is defined as an intentional state without an intentional object—that is, as a deliberate process with aversive intent which does not produce cognitive or creative objects. However, such a definition of pain surely only applies to pain that is the outcome of torture and war, where it is inflicted deliberately and is the whole point of the exercise. Such pain has social actors: political warmongers who hold state power, the military hierarchy, warlords, torturers—who have intent to maim and kill to gain territory, resources, strategic advantage, power—to silence opposition and terrorise local populations. Pain does not harbour any intention, but those who inflict it as a means to realise their ends use pain for a deliberate purpose.

Contemporary neuroscience attributes a positive function to ordinary, everyday pain as a signalling system to the brain to change course, avert danger or heal inflammation.[9] It shows this kind of pain to be a reflex reaction from local, decentred nerve endings that transmit messages in a one-way passage to the lower cortex of the brain. In the limiting case of chronic pain produced through illness or injury, the neuropathic pathways laid down appear to continue beyond any preventive or protective function, so even in metaphorical terms, pain cannot be attributed any 'intention' or 'purpose'. 'Chronic pathological pain' as defined by Cernero is a 'destructive curse'.[10] Chronic pain exerts a damaging power, capable of subjecting the individual, without prior intent or deliberative capacity. However, understood—as an early warning system to the brain, mechanically registering conflicting forces in the body, the scream of rupture of the integument of the body, permanently sensitised and altered peripheral and central neurological pathways issuing from damaged or inflamed tissue, or as a complex combination of these, even to the point of it being considered an emotion—its effects are less controversial. It is destructive of subjectivity, creativity and moral agency, tending to reduce the living self to bodily functions and repellent sensations.

Poetry and Intention

The imagination, according to Scarry, works by producing artistic objects without consciousness of the imagination as a creative process. Often visual artists articulate their work as spontaneous or intuitive—as though art comes from nowhere. Yet if we acknowledge that intuition lies at the root of all innovative endeavour—scientific as well as artistic—emerging out of deep knowledge and critical thinking that fuses in the subconscious, giving birth to new questions and insights, then we can understand why the process appears blind to its practitioners—art seen as magical, making something out of nothing. It may not be possible to define how different elements fuse—that is, the chemistry of thought, images or ideas, but you can identify a series of constituent elements that come from the culture and experience of the artist, specific moments, artistic traditions, long-term influences.

However, it is difficult to 'write about pain' intentionally because the poem resists or subverts conscious intention, working from the individual's subconscious and from the language which inescapably embodies the collective consciousness of a culture. The poem works associatively through what the language and music and form connote, through the cultural references and literary traditions it draws on, rather than just the surface content of what is denoted. In poetry it may be a line that suddenly arrives, a rhythm or an image suggested by an idea, but the writing process does not stay there as the language takes over, and in redrafting, a form or pattern of sounds and rhythms suggests itself, as though the ideal form were already there in the cultural universe, waiting to be found. In Keats's idea of 'negative capability', the poet is not only receptive to new experiences of people, places and situations (without primarily judging, rather seeking to understand them) but also open to the language—words, rhythms and patterns that lie in wait, discovering the familiar and unknown through writing and rewriting. In other words, being receptive to the possibilities of language which has its own ideas—laws, forms and music.

The danger of intentionality in communicating pain is that any message the poet wants to send in advance of writing the poem is affirming what is already known to the conscious mind and often more widely in the culture, or it appeals to a specific group. It can be said in other words and often has been—in newspaper article or political discourse. It is often stale, clichéd or lazy thought which uses the art form as a vehicle to reaffirm the virtue, justness or truth of an idea or unity of the group, reiterating for an audience who, *a priori*, agrees with the writer. This understands poetry as a form of identity politics, cheering for your own side, not as an imaginative space in which to explore and discover something previously unknown, unthought, unheard of in the language and a space also of response and interpretation by readers.

Yet against the danger of using poetry as a vehicle for reaffirming predetermined truths, it can be a valuable medium for exploring aspects of pain which are suppressed because they are difficult to address, such as the emotions of shame and self-disgust which sufferers have experienced. The carrying over of negative attributes of chronic illness and pain to the sufferers is codified in the language and culture which still influence perceptions.

The Point of Pain[11]

The master gatekeeper of the captive mind
executes both thought and generosity.
It is the body's turbine and blades that grind,
the marker mapping out anatomy—
nerve fibres, spasmic sinews, joints, inchoate
aches that heighten consciousness of the whole
and qualities of character delineate:
visceral, livy-livered, gutless, galled.
Exact and exacting in its demands, it aims
at dominion over mind and flesh and organs
it skews and stops, countered with mere half moons—
to be endured, gone through, overcome.
Once pain's rumbled, reduced to a rump, transcended
through fellow feeling, its empire's ended.

This is in sonnet form—enclosing a little argument—influenced by the metaphysical poet George Herbert's sonnet, 'Prayer' which pins down

3 An Essay on the Space Outside Pain Where the Poem Takes Place

the diverse aspects of prayer by listing its unusual and complementary attributes. My sonnet on pain tries to pin down pain in a series of material metaphors, but then invokes the negative moral qualities attributed to inner body parts in the language we have inherited from the ancient Greeks. In Galen's conception of the humours and the physiology in which they were located, the body is the location of the self and of agency, with different emotions—both virtues and vices—attached to the internal organs.[12] 'Humoral physiology' became the centre of conflict between the Church and Skeptics in early modern Europe, but both sides sought definitive proof of the soul or human character in the innards of the body. This tradition has left its traces in the language and culture, linking processes of rotting and renewal to the inner organs—a model that acupuncture shares with Shakespeare. The diseased insides were overloaded with moral connotations: the liver for cowardice, the gall bladder for bitterness, the spleen for hot-blooded impetuousness and rage. Weakness, vice and corruption have remained as powerful metaphors for the 'body politic' and the connotations have clung to the sick individual of 'feeling rotten'.

Yet Ilium, the mythic ideal city in Homer, is named after the terminal part of the small intestine. And in early modern Europe the bowels were seen as the seat of compassion by both Skeptics and the Church. Cromwell famously appealed to the Scottish Presbyterians when religious differences arose between them that undermined their previous alliance, to reconsider their position and give up their arms: 'I beseech you, in the bowels of Christ, think it possible you may be mistaken.'[13]

This more generous and accepting view of the bowels has not prevailed over the overriding connotations of baseness and defilement. The poem employs humour through euphemism and punning on *rumbling* and *rump* to allude to the unspeakable. Such discretion seeks to make the unbearable funny, and hence bearable.

Writing as a performative act enables not only mutual exploration by the writer and reader but empathy of the writer for herself/himself and for the public, by creating a space in which the difficult things—the taboo, the contradictory, confusing and unspeakable—can be shared and made lighter, if not made light of. The poem's ending suggests that empathy towards others is a way of breaking the domination of pain, connecting the sufferer's pain to that of others, so bonds are formed across pain barriers. Rather than writing as therapy—which considers pain essentially as a private matter of the individual psyche, writing as an act of empathy both to the self and to a notional public inherently involves a relationship with others, both other sufferers and the wider world of readers, audience, public culture.

Some poems show the mental process at work of moving on the skids of language where writing acts as an escape route from pain into language. The poet has to allow the process of writing itself to take the mind for a walk on an unknown path which offers a respite from the everyday reality of pain. I am totally hypnotised in suspended animation when I write, not hearing the bell ring, or the telephone, losing a sense of time, being diverted from eating, and … from pain.

Pain's Universe[14]

"God is the indwellling and not the transient cause of things."
Ethics, Baruch Spinoza (1632-77)

Recalling an uninhabited place
that no vein or membrane, organ or limb
defines, or being a part of, can embrace,
pain spreads without a centre or a rim
like the nothingness that awes a child's mind,
runs over the bounded universe of time
and all that is in it and beyond, unconfined
by the eye that cannot countenance or frame
what cause lies behind God or that there's none.
But suppose Spinoza's right and god is everywhere
in everyone, then however hard-pressing
pain cannot set us apart, for Baruch—the blessed—
shows another way of seeing, that in the sheer
boundlessness of space we are not alone.

This poem enacts a chain of thought—which subverts the isolating effects of actual pain. Not consciously setting out to write about pain, the cosmological metaphor 'came to me', as did the whole poem, bar the epigraph, ready-formed with all the rhymes. Its landscape suggests an immensity of scale—of pain without boundaries, linked to the child's disturbing experience of being transported away by thinking of infinity …. The language is hieratic and informal in turn, going from philosophical speculation to a homely thought experiment to a consoling idea as the mind unreels. Likewise it starts with the boundless power of pain as a kind of parallel, monotheistic omnipotent God—beyond any local sensory understanding, without discernible cause, almost beyond human comprehension but through following a thought process arrives at a pantheistic sense of the human spirit not as unknowable and external, but personal and universal.

By creating imaginative objects that convey or represent pain, or its effects, by giving it objective correlatives in the imaginative world, the interiority of pain and the isolation of the chronic pain sufferer find external expression that maybe even recast pain and so diminish its power over the person. The poem transforms the originating impulse, but is not reducible to the origin (sick person) or surface theme, (pain, cosmology) or just individual experience (autobiography of being kept awake as a child by wondering what was beyond the edge of the universe). Part of the liberation of writing is that the poem transforms the intention of the sufferer and may take her/him somewhere else. Language allows the writer to travel and transcend so poet and reader/audience learn something surprising from a turn in the direction of a poem. The main purpose of writing a poem is not to confirm what the poet already knows but to discover something that s/he did not know—or even that s/he did not know they knew that could not be put into any other words or form of discourse. Why otherwise a poem on pain rather than a treatise or newspaper article or the spoken word?

Metaphors of Pain

By creating imaginative objects that convey or represent pain and its effects through art, finding objective correlatives in the real world, the interiority of pain finds external expression. It is precisely because pain has no immediate material referents in the real world and the science remains hazy about the connections between pain signals and how the brain interprets and processes them where they appear without any preventive or protective function, that pain can only be represented through metaphor—imagining objects which evoke through association its qualities, attributes and effects.

Sontag in *Illness as Metaphor* writes a powerful critique of metaphors of war and 'fighting' disease—particularly emblematic diseases such as cancer and AIDS—that stigmatise the sufferers along with the illness, as responsible, through their reprehensible behaviour, for their condition. She shows how these illnesses are used as metaphors for the body politic, national character and foreign invaders, reinforcing a nationalist, militarist narrative of the disease. By contrast, she suggests a healthy way of being ill—at least with cancer—is to resist metaphoric thinking. In the process of arguing for knowledge of cancer as an illness, stripped of metaphors of evil and malignancy, she comes close to arguing for scientific knowledge and rationality without culture, for discussion of these illnesses without cultural representations of them. Although she acknowledges that metaphors are essential for thought, she seeks to be rid of militarist ones. While the overall argument is persuasive against stereotypical racist, nationalist and bellicose representations of these diseases, it is not conceivable to give up metaphors of conflict, struggle and defeat of chronic illness and pain.

How can pain be imaginatively transformed by the sufferer without conflictual metaphors? How can pain be reconceived without it being seen as an enemy? There is no pain or illness without social contexts within which it is treated, without living sufferers trying to hold on to their bombarded subjectivity and the conflicting emotions which severe and persistent illness and pain throw up; without cultural representations of pain and illness in the way they are written about and framed, including by scientists. Therefore, they are never scientific without also being cultural constructs, and inevitably metaphoric. The question is how precise, how truthful, how meaningful, how beneficial are the metaphors? Where Sontag argues illness is real and not metaphorical, and not a war this is not overly helpful. For years, my own disease was not treated as 'real' and it came as a relief when finally it was diagnosed, given a name and some kind of treatment although without much clarity over causes or cure. So I empathise with the desire to pin a disease down, ascertain its scientific status and treatment, even though science is imagined as being neutral, rational and outside culture, and illness as being located in the body without complicated feedback mechanisms from the body to the brain and emotions and the mind to the body. But I cannot conceive metaphors of chronic illness and pain which are benign or devoid of conflict. While Sontag makes a convincing case against the use of metaphors of war on diseases for macho nationalistic purposes, chronic illness and pain remain aversive and hostile to the body and self.

So you cannot make friends with chronic pain. You can only passively accept it or fight it, not with weapons of militarism in a war of attrition, but more appropriately in 'a war of position', to borrow Gramsci's term, by winning support in all the instances of public mobilisation, communication and influence, winning support through persuasion, refusing isolation and silence, to outwit and outmanoeuvre the enemy. This means deploying different weapons in self-defence, rather than retaliatory violence, but it does mean real defence of the self through the imagination, through building relationships with others to break the isolation, through subversive challenge and contestation. The struggle with chronic illness and pain is between life forces and energies which are in contest for control. Perhaps the most exact metaphor is that of resistance, first of all refusing passive acceptance of a brutal regime and mobilising moral and mental resources to take solidaristic action.

The metaphors in these poems on pain range widely: in 'Crohn heroine' a sense of an interior enemy which has created a wasteland, a wreck of a rusting body, violent explosions and devastation; in 'Reflection' an echo of the Holocaust in fear of the showerhead and of disappearing flesh, but counteracted by holding on to the mind, to memory, to the present. In 'Pain's Universe' the cosmological and geological metaphors are subordinate to the enactment of the mind running away with itself to outwit pain. The industrial machinery and energy production in 'The Point of Pain' stand for how pain reproduces its dominance; the awful offal embody both self-disgust and the moral taint in the language of diseased or deficient internal organs. It also shifts to political metaphor, but the explicit opposite of militarism, in its imagined defeat of empire and end of domination through empathy and solidarity.

Passage from Pain to the Political

The passage from pain to the political is a path from passive subordinate to active subject, marked by the experience of chronic illness but not consumed or defined by it alone. It entails redefining subjectivity, reclaiming the self as a thinking being with moral and political agency, while at the same time recognising interdependency and what is universal even in the most specific, intimate and ineffable of experiences.

It is the premise of my poems that, through empathy, they can reach the reader who has not experienced chronic pain. This entails decentering the self, even if it begins with autobiography. The question is how does it connect to others, how does it make it imaginable to those who have not been through the same experience? That depends on the efficacy of the metaphor and music, the emotional connection, the persuasiveness of the thought. If it is authentic, can it also conjure up other kinds of pain or violence legitimately without demeaning the scale and significance of that greater historic suffering?

Toast

> Wanting the bronze tinge of cinnamon
> the porous surface letting in the butter
> that slips through, seeps and moistens
> I grab at the drying bread under the grill
> and get baked hand with crisped
> red-brown skin, lashings of screaming
> a thick layer of Savlon cream
> and the tight raw feeling of being ironed.
> Dr. Marcus bribes me with a sweet
> to tear the stuck gauze off and underneath:
> the dried lands of Relleu[15] and the Jordan valley.

In the poem the metaphor of a hand being burnt to a crisp and skin being ironed are extended to the desiccation of land in Spain and the Jordan Valley and maybe a hint of people being roasted alive in the Middle East. As we operate within culture and language as a social, cognitive and imaginative construct, it is possible for the poem to work beyond the bounds of essential origins, and resound with wider allusions that the language carries, including those the reader brings to it.

The paradox remains that the poet needs to fight for her/his subjectivity against pain while at the same time diminishing ego so it does not get in the way of the poem and its effective communication … so it works as art. I want recognition of my suffering and struggle, at the same time as not being subsumed or defined by them. I need also to be part of something bigger than myself but at the same time that recognises my specific voice, marked by that experience, that I carry the scars and pain with me. There is no pure unsullied self and perhaps that is true of everyone …. This poem addresses some of the ambivalence of living with chronic pain and with wider forms of domination. It came out of a Communicating Chronic Pain workshop which formed part of the fruitful exchange between artists, neuroscientists and clinicians that the project made possible:

If not for this[16]

The man introduced himself as an Alexander practitioner of the art of aligning the body as perfectly as it once was before contorted with pain. *Me is me* he said … *there is the me before pain, outside of pain, you know this.* We had to scrape around inside ourselves to find any point of contact with the absurdist notion of choice … even more with the idea we might exist in a free republic outside the empire of pain, and anyway some of us were proud to have learnt hypersensitivity from the brawl and squall of it. Who would we be if not for this? Where would we be without the resilience of our scars, our terrors, our reason?

Notes

1. Sontag, Susan. *Illness as Metaphor and Aids and Its Metaphors* (Penguin, 1991, 2002), p. 3.
2. "Pain – has an Element of Blank." In *The Poems of Emily Dickinson*, edited by Thomas A. Johnson (Belknap Press, 1955).
3. "There is a pain so utter," Johnson ed. ibid.

4. Department of Work and Pensions, *Mortality Statistics: Employment and Support Allowance, Incapacity Benefit or Severe Disability Allowance*, August 2015, p. 8.
5. Sontag, Susan. *Regarding the Pain of Others* (Penguin, 2004), p. 20.
6. Published in *Envoi*, 172, February 2016, p. 31.
7. Recorded as a backdrop to the hospital video by Richard Crow for desperate optimists, which was later used in the Communicating Chronic Pain workshop on sound.
8. Scarry, Elaine. *The Body in Pain. The Making and Unmaking of the World* (New York; Oxford: Oxford University Press, 1985).
9. Fernando Cervero, *Understanding Pain*, (Massachusetts: MIT Press, 2014) on the nociceptors or 'good pain' which is protective.
10. Ibid., p. 11, 73.
11. Published in the pamphlet *A Small Gateway*, Jude Rosen (Hearing Eye, 2009).
12. Hillman, David. "Visceral Knowledge, Shakespeare, Skepticism and the Interior of the Early Modern Body." In *The Body in Parts: Fantasies of Corporeality in Early Modern Europe*, edited by Hillman David and Mazzio Carla (New York; London: Routledge, 1997), p. 82.
13. Oliver Cromwell, Letter to the General Assembly of the Church of Scotland, 3 August 1650.
14. Published in the pamphlet *A Small Gateway*, Jude Rosen (Hearing Eye, 2009).
15. A village in the Valencian mountains which has lost its water.
16. Published in *Envoi*, 172, February 2016, p. 16.

Jude Rosen is an independent urban researcher and poet, translator and former lecturer in modern European studies at UCL until ill-health retirement. Her poetry pamphlet *A Small Gateway* (Hearing Eye, 2009) included sonnets on pain, and other poems on pain were published in *Envoi*, 2016. Since 2007, she has been writing a poetry collection on the Olympic zone and marshlands of the Lower Lea Valley, *Reclamations*, (forthcoming 2018) an urban pastorale of encroachment on wild spaces and displacement of people, performed on 'poem and living history walks' of the area.

4

Act Like It Hurts: Questions of Role and Authenticity in the Communication of Chronic Pain

Sarah Goldingay

Playing Doctors and Patients

This chapter will use the lenses of performance and culture to explore the significance of role and authenticity in the communication of chronic pain. It sets out to better understand some challenges of this communication process created by cultural archetypes and their associated tropes. The archetypes it examines are the culturally naturalised[1] roles of Doctor and Patient.[2] It explores how the role of 'indestructible' Doctor provides a counterpoint to that of the 'fragile' Patient. It examines how these roles become shorthand, *personae*, for the people taking part in the human-to-human interactions that form healthcare interventions. Noting Talcott Parsons' problematic identification of the so-called *sick role*,[3] and that these roles offer a useful starting point to set out the social contracts[4] and normative behaviours that characterise a Doctor–Patient interaction, their fixity and binary nature can limit the development of the relationship over time. The perceived authenticity of the Doctor–Patient relationship is central to healing.[5]

S. Goldingay (✉)
University of Exeter, Exeter, UK

As a Patient moves towards better health or finds a way of flourishing with their chronic condition, they are no longer 'fragile'. If they are no longer fragile, then how does the role of Doctor shift in response? In an exploration of the Aristotelian idea of flourishing, Hope May observes, '"happiness" denotes an emotional state that comes and goes, flourishing denotes something deeper, more permanent: Think: *awakening, enlightenment or self-actualization*'.[6] We might also say that health is a state that comes and goes. If a person is to flourish, empowered to self-actualise, regardless of their state of health, then the fixed role of the fragile patient cannot serve them for very long.[7] Yet, this role of fragility is culturally dominant. Through the encounters of their everyday lives, this is the cultural trope people—who find themselves in the role of Patient—are invited to identify with and play against. In a conversation, Pete Moore, inspiring public speaker and developer of the popular online resource *The Pain Toolkit*,[8] underlined the imaginative potency of the role of the fragile patient. As someone living with chronic pain for several years, he pointed out that even with all his experience and understanding of how to live well with a chronic condition, when faced with a new illness he immediately shifted out of the driving seat of his life. Pete explained that he had let the physicians take over not only the driving but also the route planning and even identifying the destination of his healing journey. Only when he reminded himself that he spends on average three hours a year with healthcare professionals and the rest of the time he was necessarily drawing on his own resources did he get back behind the steering wheel.[9] Pete advocates a process of awakening people with chronic pain from their role of fragile patient to become self-actualised through self-management. He, in a very real sense, becomes a role model. As the chapter unfolds, we will return to this idea and examine what this new understanding of flourishing with chronic pain might be and how that possibility throws light on how these roles operate within broader cultural tropes. First, I want to turn our attention from the role of Patient to the role of Doctor.

Doctors also find their life experience does not always align with their understanding of their given role of 'indestructible' Doctor. Despite the traits of authority, competence and congruence that dominate cultural descriptions, Doctors, in reality, are not indestructible; they too are patients; they too question their knowledge, and they too are frustrated by their inability to cure. As one rheumatologist I interviewed explained, feelings of *unease and uncertainty often characterised his* experience of treating patients. He felt untrained for this emotional response:

> In our business, we Doctors don't pay attention to what an encounter makes us feel. We sit in an analytical frame of mind, trying to figure out what the diagnosis might be, which drug to give, etc., while the patient weeps quietly in the other corner of the room. We may worry about what they are feeling, but we never stop to consider what we are feeling ourselves.[10]

In our conversation, this Doctor described an incongruence in his understanding: when he was meeting with people with osteoarthritis and chronic pain, he had a set of expectations. Often these were implicit, based on what dominant culture led him to expect; sometimes they were burnished by his training. Yet, repeatedly, his expectations were overturned by his experiences. He built his understanding of his role of Doctor, in the given context of a consultation, on the expectation that cure would inevitably follow the correct process—analysis, diagnosis, prescription. However, this, in his experience, was not enough. In the years leading up to his retirement, without being able to offer a cure, he increasingly relied on care. Care for his patients, and for himself. He noted that the dominant culture of medicine does not allow for self-reflection and flourishing for Doctors; this is rejected, pejoratively, as a matter of 'navel gazing'.[11] Yet, the Doctor also needs to flourish, to move beyond the fixity of a role to enable *awakening, enlightenment or self-actualization.*[12] This sense of self-worth, of self-care, matters, both in terms of avoiding so-called burn-out and ensuring practitioner retention.

Under scrutiny, neither the role of Doctor nor Patient is fixed. They are placeholders in evolving social contracts. These contracts are enacted within social encounters—stories and tropes. These narrative constructs offer good ways to think about how these archetypal roles shift over time and within context. This chapter will examine how those experiencing chronic pain and those setting out to understand and care for another with chronic pain might share the same stories but not share experiences or meanings in the interpretation of those stories. I will examine why, despite this common beginning, chronic pain is hard to describe and, in its reception and interpretation, even harder to understand. I will also consider the converse of this culture-creates-experience cycle by examining not only the ways in which stories undermine the authenticity of a patient's claims of illness and pain but also the ways that wider societal structures are responding to the rise in chronic conditions. In its theoretical underpinnings, the chapter is interdisciplinary. It draws on three key areas. From medicine, it uses neuro-regulatory theory and the placebo response to think about the impact meaning-making and context has on wellbeing. From psychology, it draws on studies centred on validation and invalidation to examine how the way that we interpret interactions impacts on our health, and from theatre, drama and performance studies, I use scholarship concerned with communication and reception theories and the relationship of cultural formation to somatic experiences.

Acute Stories in a Chronic World

Stories not only describe a Doctor–Patient interaction but also a much larger context. Cultural tropes overlap to frame the healthcare consultation with the wider concepts of health, wellbeing and the healthcare system. The dominant narratives about healthcare presented by popular culture are increasingly redundant in the face of rising chronic conditions, especially in the communication of chronic pain. Stories of acute conditions dominate. For example, the BBC television show *Casualty* has been running in a prime-time slot for more than 30 years. Each week it has millions of viewers. The drama is set in an acute hospital where somatic damage, trauma caused by events like a road traffic accident, is successfully treated. Each week patients are restored to their previous state of health, often receive some sort of psychological healing or reconciliation, and leave not only bodily cured but also made whole emotionally and spiritually. Patients, who only appear in one show to enable the episodic format, leave cured, never to return. To sustain interest, characters who continue throughout the series, the healthcare professionals, are flawed in some way. These flaws are not, in dramaturgical terms, fatal flaws. These are ones the audience can imagine in themselves through a cathartic engagement, mirroring their own flaws. Resolving the characters' flaws offers a different kind of slow-burning drama; the structure of the dramatic arc needs character development to sustain audience engagement. However, while we may see these characters have ongoing challenges in their love lives or relationships with their colleagues, there is never any questioning of their ability to act with unfailing integrity and unquestionable knowledge in relationship to their patients. The reason I offer this example is that to be successful any dramatic form needs conflict; it needs it change and needs it a resolution. Acute medicine too follows this form. Therefore, the stories told about medicine in popular culture are typically acute. There is trauma, followed by treatment and cure. Moreover, as these fictional stories bleed into our real lives, these dominant tropes sustain nostalgia for a once experienced, healthier past and a romanticised golden age of healthcare. They not only make the stories we tell ourselves, but they are already made of the stories we have told ourselves. They shape our expectations about our own recovery from illness; we expect to have acute conditions and swift, permanent cures delivered by an indestructible Doctor. In reality, however, chronic conditions now dominate.[13] Many people cannot be cured of common long-term conditions and their associated chronic pain.

Healthcare is heterogeneous, but we tend to use binary oppositions to frame it: 'Is a person "well" or "ill"? Are they a doctor or a patient, for example?' One such binary is acute versus chronic medicine. Although this offers a useful shorthand, in actuality there is a continuum. At its extreme ends are two different models: the acute interventional one, and the chronic care model. Epitomised by emergency room medicine, critical care, resuscitation and surgery, the acute interventional type forms the dramatic storylines for a television show like *Casualty*: It is about making quick decisions about how to save life or limb. The healthcare revolution and its success has been predicated on an acute model of healthcare delivery and the biomedical model of disease—the concept that reductionist science can find the causes of diseases, and hence ways of curing them. The limitations of a theory based on cellular and molecular science, and on one way of knowing, have been acknowledged by many critics of modern medicine[14] and will not be pursued further here. While it dominates culturally and in practice, acute medicine is only part of the story. The chronic care model is different. It is about helping people with chronic health problems who do not require any immediate intervention, but who are explicitly looking for appropriate advice and perhaps, more importantly, for understanding from others. However, ill people do not always sit at these extremes, and indeed a single case may move its position over time, and a person may have both acute and chronic conditions simultaneously. Unfortunately, Western healthcare infrastructures do not explicitly recognise these differences or these overlaps. Similarly, healthcare professionals interact with patients without distinguishing clearly enough between these two polar extremes—or understanding the importance of the relations between them. Later in the chapter, I will use my experience of teaching in a medical school and feedback gained from the students I was teaching to think about how they, with a little encouragement, can recognise the need to distinguish between modes of medicine for themselves despite the limitations of their syllabus. Encouragingly, they are already able to reflect on the dynamic nature of their role in a system that is changing. There are few aspects of culture that tell this chronic story. And yet we live in stories; they help us understand our experience of the world. Therefore, different stories need to be told to help people with chronic pain understand themselves and the significant change they are encountering in their lives.

Performance and Medicine

When I encounter people from other disciplines, they most often ask me how theatre can help us better understand wellbeing and healing. I usually say that I look through the 'lens of performance' to find a new understanding about how context effects wellbeing. However, this is far from simple. In medicine, the term 'performance' most often makes reference to an outcome that is measured against an established scale, whereas for performance studies it is chameleon-like[15]: It might be analysis of a new piece of theatre about chronic pain[16] or a better understanding of how culture shapes—and is shaped by—the way we think about being old and getting older as a society.[17] It is not always about exploring something that is explicitly 'a performance'. Its methods and modes are also used beyond theatre buildings to examine everyday life 'as if' it is a performance.[18] A performance-led approach is longitudinal, contextual and systemic: performance is a network of things made meaningful—the lens of performance is a means of describing, analysing and reflecting on human interactions that set out to create change in a context that shifts over time.

The anthropological 'turn' in performance studies, which developed out of the work of researcher-practitioners such as Schechner and Turner,[19] has thrown light on the way in which all kinds of societies, from the tribal to the urban-industrial, use performance to effect change in the real world. Combined with a semiotics of theatre and everyday life,[20] it demonstrates how the performances of, for example, the church or the courtroom can be analysed in terms of costumes, scripts, sets, rituals and narrative structures.[21] Medical practice, also, can be analysed in these terms. The theatre in which a surgeon performs is analogous to that in which an actor performs. Elsewhere the Doctor, carrying props and wearing costumes that signify purity, knowledge and power (the stethoscope and white coat, or more typically now a computer and scrubs), asks questions that follow a pre-existing script shaped by the medical profession's well-established system of 'taking a patient history'. The *mise-en-scène* is often a consulting room where both Doctor and Patient play roles that are societally prescribed. In this space with special healing significance, they take part in shared rituals, set apart in space and time. These rituals also extend into the patient's everyday life through stage directions for a new ritual to be embodied three times daily through ingestion or application.

The insight that medical practice can be seen as a kind of everyday performance will be of interest in itself to some people. Certainly, it is the sort of provocation that is useful in teaching undergraduates on performance studies programmes to think more broadly about what we understand by the concept of 'performance'. However, then the question arises, 'So what?' What implications, if any, can be drawn from such an insight? More specifically, are there any implications that might have value for the practice of medicine? To set up the framework for this discussion, I will start with some theatre history and a now legendary event.

The Imaginary Invalid

We are in Paris, at the theatre in the late afternoon of February 17th, 1673. Notable French playwright and actor, Molière is on stage. He is playing the part of the hypochondriac, Argan, in his celebrated play *Le Malade Imaginaire [The Imaginary Invalid]*. The play is also known, in other translations, as *The Hypochondriac*. In setting out to understand the role of both Patient and Doctor, the idea of the hypochondriac matters. We may be considering a play written almost 400 years ago, but it still has cultural currency today. Not only has it been translated into several languages, but also it continues to be regularly performed, audiences still buy tickets to see it, and it is still included as a key text in educational syllabi. While any claims for universality are not borne out in the detail of individual interpretation, the wide-spread appeal and sustained success of this play that suggests an ongoing engagement with its themes because they speak to a shared experience of what it is to be human. *The Imaginary Invalid* is a three-act comédie-ballet with dance sequences and musical interludes. The comedy of Moliere's play can only work because this is a deep-seated cultural trope shared by the audience, writer and actors. The hypochondriac, as an archetype, is a cluster of cultural narratives and norms that have coalesced to become a stock character, one to be repeated across times and cultures, and importantly for us, become naturalised. These are ideas that are accepted and are so commonplace as to be beyond question. These archetypes, like those of the hypochondriac, are seldom problematised in our everyday life; they are a convenient shorthand that helps us understand the world.

As intelligent individuals, when we are invited to reconsider these naturalised ideas directly we do problematise them, challenge them and reconsider them. However, this invitation is not common and any person setting out to communicate their experience of chronic pain is always playing against this shorthand. If we consider the Doctor–Patient interaction as if it is a performance—longitudinal, contextual and systemic: a network of things made meaningful—then what is the patient setting out to do in their part of this interaction? At the moment when the Doctor asks how they can help, first, the Patient always needs to demonstrate, on some level, that they are not a hypochondriac, that their pain is real, unpredictable and persistent. Second, the person with pain needs to problematise the archetype of the hypochondriac for the individual they are speaking with; regardless of how aware and sensitive the Doctor, they too are culturally constructed and doubting the authenticity of the presenting pain is part of their role. Third and simultaneously, the Patient also needs to problematise the role of hypochondria for themselves—still, the notion persists that it is 'all in the mind', non-material, and despite pain's somatic manifestation is, therefore, inauthentic and fraudulent. Fourth, in the moment of trying to understand their experience of persistent pain while interpreting their own encounter in a context of acute cure and trying to second-guess and interpret the Doctor's response, the Patient is simultaneously setting out to communicate an experience that is very real to them but often beyond words. This experience is usually beyond understanding and typically beyond the credulity given by a textbook pathology.[22] Fifth, this communication is not only taking place in the moment of face-to-face dialogue but is also informed by the past. It is a coalescence of a number of interpretations of selves and roles and experiences and understandings that do not, necessarily, agree within the Patient's current sense of self. Sixth, this complexity is compounded when we note that the person they are speaking with is also tumbling through their own interpretative process: the Doctor is encountering the chronic in an acute trope that is explicitly expressed in both the healthcare environment and the wider dominant culture. Both Doctor and Patient are setting out to engage with the imagination and understanding of the other in a context-dependant encounter. As they shift together, over time, they attempt to communicate and interpret an experience of a past-tense body that was free of pain and a present-tense body in pain. Pain is notoriously difficult to understand, and we set out to understand it in a dominant cultural trope that does not fully allow for the idea of the chronic.[23] No wonder then that communication around chronic pain is difficult. To examine the complexity of the Doctor–Patient exchange further, let us return to Moliere's performance of a hypochondriac because his creation and performance of *The Imaginary Invalid* is not as straightforward as simply the playing of an archetype to make an audience laugh.

The 'Real' Actor

In the late afternoon of a Paris winter, we continue to watch Moliere's fourth performance of *The Imaginary Invalid*, and we have seen his character of Argan test the patience and credulity of his family, staff and doctors who are treating his nebulous malady, and its shifting symptoms. As we observe, something extraordinary begins to happen. Moliere, the actor, begins to cough. He has been coughing for weeks and suffering from poor health for some time. An actor, who despite failing health, insisted earlier that day he must continue to work. Famously he states that many mouths rely on his work; we might now see why this is such an important idea for Moliere's biographers because it is a clear expression of the popular trope told about theatrical performers, 'the show must go on'. Similar stories are also told about the admirable qualities of the 'indestructible' Doctors. This event is his fourth and final performance of Argan; Moliere dies soon after this performance ends. The actor is not then the hypochondriac; he is the hero, the martyr perhaps. Paradoxically, he is playing a character, a hypochondriac, who is feigning poor physical health. At this moment, we can begin to see how multiple roles and experiences can occupy the same space simultaneously. Reality and make-believe are not an easy binary that offer a clean taxonomy of how the world works, but rather porous categories of understanding and experience. In his performance, Moliere as actor and character is both authentic and inauthentic, well and ill. In this multi-phrenic state,[24] he offers a means for us to reconsider the binary of the Doctor–Patient relationship. In their embodiment of both or either role, people can express both potentials. Even though the Patient's pain is real, they have no means to demonstrate it materially. Moreover, while the Doctor believes their patient, they have no ways to describe it pathologically.

Cultural approaches that draw on stereotypical assumptions about health and illness, symptom and cure do not account for the complexity of chronic pain, where experiences are far from linear, often opaque and notoriously difficult to communicate. The implications of that shift from acute to chronic medicine and associated conditions demand new kinds of cultural understanding of, and assumptions about, pain. Yet, in terms of cultural representation, there is a time lag: we have not caught up yet. That 'we' includes not just the general public and popular culture but medical practitioners too. In 1951 Talcott Parsons developed the term *sick role* to describe a pattern of behaviour—a cultural role—adopted by someone who is sick. By later extension, this came to describe someone who does not have a 'real' illness but has chosen to perform a 'role' in order to exempt themselves from the responsibilities of everyday life. They are then 'acting sick' and consequently should be understood as hypochondriacs, malingerers and frauds: thus the social stereotype and theatrical stock character—the hypochondriac—becomes mobilised as a diagnostic category.

Things have moved on in medical practice since 1951; a more nuanced and empathetic approach is in evidence. Even so, for the patient, the experience of chronic pain is often hard to articulate, and for the physician, it is hard to understand. In the philosophy of medicine, this is called 'the problem of the other mind'. This approach recognises we cannot know what someone else is experiencing and this makes a diagnosis and treatment difficult. It assumes no two experiences of pain are the same; the patient can complain of pain without having any and can have pain without complaining. In this complex converse perception, the genuinely sick person pretends that their complaint is unimportant, or less severe, to perform the role of martyr, hero or heroine. Whether heroine or hypochondriac or more likely somewhere in between, the onus of responsibility falls to the Patient to convince the Doctor of the truth of their experience. They need to find a way of convincing the Doctor of their own authenticity, to demonstrate they are not acting. Which makes the point is that we need to move beyond the simple binary opposition of 'genuinely sick' versus 'malingerer'.

Performance studies can help here. Theatrical performance has always raised questions about authenticity and inauthenticity. Undergraduates are invited to think about everyday life 'as if' it is a performance. Before turning the methods and modes of performance analysis to the outside world, they typically begin by learning about more straightforward theatrical analysis. These are approaches that turn around textual analysis, a close reading of the script; semiotics to help them analyse the materiality of the setting; the mode or genre of the performance, the tradition that it best fits; and a poststructural analytical frame, such as postcolonialism or feminism. However, in the liveness of the performance, when the script is enacted by bodies moving in real space and time for an audience who are interpreting their encounter individually and collectively, analysis becomes challenging. We ask them to explain how in the auditorium, a space of artifice, filled with someone saying prewritten words who is pretending to be someone else can change an audience member's understanding of the world. We might ask, how can make-believe make belief? How can the inauthentic bring about authentic change? In theatre analysis, provisionality, interpretation and subjectivity are central; there are no absolutes but rather a set of continuums. On such a continuum, the binary oppositions of authentic and inauthentic become unhelpful. They are instead markers of interpretation. So, what about what happens in the consulting room? How can something as transitory and provisional as long-term pain be expressed in a way that is readily understood by a system of pathology? How can the Patient who has little material evidence of their persistent, life-changing pain convince the Doctor of the authenticity of their experience when it does not fit the dominant narrative of acute medicine? We need to offer different tropes that contain more fluid roles.

In the next section, recognising the important work being done around 'The Hidden Curriculum',[25] I use some teaching I did with medical students to explore how current cultural narratives within medical education set up the pursuit of a particular understanding of the role of the authentic Doctor. I throw light on how current medical students are being taught apparently innate communication skills such as empathy and conclude by considering the importance of an empathetic capacity in light of new research around the placebo response.

Performing Both Patient and Doctor

The use of traditional theatre forms to help medical students think about the need for flexible modes of communication offers a helpful starting point to consider how the tropes of acute medicine and medical training shape the experience of people with chronic pain. In collaboration with a colleague from the medical school, I gave an interactive, performative lecture to the whole of the first year ($n = 130$). We provided an opening context that scaffolded onto students' pre-existing knowledges and expectations. We highlighted their experiences as patients and their existing capacity as human beings to have successful human-to-human interactions. We then gave them a short script representing a medical consultation.

> *PATIENT*: I've been feeling under the weather.
> *DOCTOR*: I'm sorry to hear that.

Two volunteers enacted the script for the whole group. As facilitators, we then took a step back and invited students to intervene and reshape the interaction. We used techniques drawn from Augusto Boal's method of Forum Theatre which grew from a desire to address socio-political inequality. Forum Theatre has a clear form and rules of engagement: actors perform a short scripted play, the subject matter of which is of immediate relevance to the audience.

> Typically the plot involves a protagonist experiencing some [...] social oppression or obstacle which s/he is unable to overcome. After this first showing of the play [there is a] short discussion with the audience about the issues facing the protagonist. The play is then played over again, but with an important difference: during this second performance, whenever an audience member feels the protagonist might usefully have tried a different strategy, s/he can stop the action, take the protagonist's place, and try out his or her idea. The other actors, who are playing the oppressors, will improvise their reactions to this new strategy, trying to maintain the oppression and attempting to bring events to their original ending. Any number of interventions can be made. Sometimes a new strategy will succeed, sometimes it will fail, or be judged unrealistic by the rest of the audience, but in either case the improvisations attempt to deal realistically with them. Forum Theatre demonstrates the number of alternative possibilities, in which strategies for responding to and changing that situation are explored, rehearsed and enacted. A successful Forum Theatre event offers an audience a sense of agency, community and empowerment.[26]

The key ideas, then, to distil from that description of Forum Theatre are its repetition, that it has no official end point, there is no one way of doing it, it is democratic, it values the participant's pre-existing life experience and it is empowering.

The students then spent an hour working through different possibilities as pairs, small groups and a whole cohort. The words remained the same—they followed the same script, but most other things changed: they tested out architectural configurations—moving desks and chairs; interior design—closing blinds and doors, using screens to hide and reveal images; they tried different emotions—the way they said the words, what their bodies showed; they shifted tone—playing hurried versus capacious consultations; they explored timing—how long they took before making eye contact, the distance and therefore the walking time from the door to the desk; they eventually tried silence—seen as particularly difficult; they tested different proxemics of the relationship—from sitting on each other's laps to sitting at either end of the lecture theatre. This was a systemic, not reductionist approach. They understood how all of these elements combined and shifted over time and context: inside the permission of the performance form they were able to see the consultation as a network of things made meaningful. Through the process, they were able to refine the performed consultation that they saw their peers act out in an effort to improve the quality of communication in the Doctor–Patient interaction. However, more importantly, as they took turns to be both Doctor and Patient under the direction of their peers, they felt emotions in response to the encounter. They identified and burnished their own pre-existing experiences of empathy and built a portfolio of experiences for future encounters.

In a focus group held the following week, the consensus was that this valuing of their pre-existing empathetic skills was 'surprisingly empowering'. The role of Doctor is a privileged social figure. Its authority carries weight in our cultural narratives, not needing to be further 'empowered'; this also includes the medical student. They do not appear to be very representative of 'the oppressed' for whom Freire, and then Boal, first developed their politicised theatrical practices.[27] However, their experience of education and medical training offers limited opportunity flourish, especially if we return to May's earlier definition of flourishing as an *awakening, enlightenment or self-actualization*. Power structures and oppression operate in multiple ways. As first noted in the *Boys in White*,[28] medical education is about enculturation into passive acceptance of the existing model of healthcare. Therefore, medical education is, in no small part, about integrating the next generation into the logic of the present system. It is about learning to embody and enact the role of Doctor, rather than about the practice of personal freedom. It is, therefore, oppressive rather than liberating, about controlling and modifying pre-existing behaviour.

In our work with the students, knowledge-as-experience came up against knowledge as validated by a hierarchical authority. When speaking about her experience, one student reflected:

> It made me rethink my professional practice work [and...] made me want to get up and change the real consultations that I've been observing. [...] You had us work things out for ourselves. You didn't tell us if something was good or bad.[29]

What is for performance specialists a simple Forum Theatre structure, used as a political device in some settings, a rehearsal technique for others, opened up new and complex perceptions for medical students. This experience was not about taking a patient history or diagnosis, but rather about the consultation process itself, about the reflexive capacity of the Doctor to be self-empowered. It also raised questions about the ways that, within a resolutely hierarchical knowledge framework, apparently, innate capacities such as empathy can be taught or controlled.[30]

Another student described a tension she identified after the session between different types of knowledge as experience and the value of its source. When describing the way that empathy is taught in medical school, she noted:

> They (the approved words...) are not yours. They make you sound robotic. They should be a way into a structure, not a fixed script.[31]

In medical training, empathy has value. Without that value, it would not be included in the packed curriculum of the Medical School. However, for it to meet the logic of the system, it must be measurable, repeatable. Consequently, it is reduced to a checklist and approved phrases. The production of a script gives empathy authenticity. However, in the live performance of the Doctor–Patient consultation, it becomes inauthentic—it is not sufficiently responsive to a context-dependent encounter that shifts over time. Without claiming that empathy is universally present, the inherent social skills a student arrives at their training with is overturned by the authority of the system they are entering. In this way, their pre-existing, cultural understanding of the role of Doctor is overturned by the role as defined by medical training. This hierarchical inversion does not aid flourishing.

This student's personal experience is symptomatic of a broader and more deeply rooted problem—the trope which both Doctors and Patients find themselves in runs counter to their embodied experience of how to communicate well, with care and empathy. The role they are trying to perform is often one they are not well qualified to play, nor appropriate for the encounter they find themselves in; it is inauthentic.

Authentically Empathetic?

There has been much research on the importance of compassion and empathy in healthcare encounters.[32] Much of the neurobiology of empathy is concerned with mirror neurons (the system that facilitates imitation of the gestures of others).[33] Physician empathy has been defined as the understanding of the patient as well as verbal and nonverbal communications that result in changes in patient behaviour[34]; this definition views empathy as the creation of a relationship that facilitates appropriate use of treatments. The creation of a good relationship can go beyond facilitating the use of treatments to enable whole person healing. Empathy goes further still. At the heart of it is the physician's capacity to be 'present' with their patient.[35] In terms of medical training and patient care, Carl Rogers' theory about the importance of clinical behaviour remains important.[36] He suggested that to be an effective clinician was to be genuine, display positive regard, show unconditional regard and be empathic. A four-level framework describes therapeutic 'presence' as presence, partial presence, full presence, and transcendental presence.[37] From a common-sense perspective, this is unsurprising: Our life experience repeatedly demonstrates that some people help us feel better, others do not. As we have already seen, empathy training has been introduced into some medical schools; however, in this context the human interaction of the consultation is often reduced to a script. As a result, the words spoken are no longer 'genuine' because they are not the clinician's own and do not arise from the current consultation. In some way their life experience, what they know to be authentic, is not present with them in the encounter.

An empathic encounter invites both Doctor and Patient to draw on the well-honed social skills they already have to shape the bio-medical trope they are in. However, the structure of the dominant trope, with its sustained drive towards reproducibility, short timeframes and litigious protectionism does not allow for the full range of that human expertise to be valued or expressed. In this way, neither Doctor nor Patient can flourish, as they are not empowered to self-actualise. Each is focused on finding the inauthentic in the other's story and enactment of their role; yet without a sense of authenticity no matter how empathetic the other is intending to be, it cannot be interpreted as such. In an inauthentic encounter, one cannot feel safe.

The way that we interpret context affects our health, healing and flourishing. This can be for better and for worse. For people with chronic pain, the healthcare encounter is often negative. They feel invalidated, unheard, a waste of space. As one woman explained to me:

> It was the third time I'd been to see my GP and I felt bad going again but I had to do something. I couldn't work. I'm a cleaner and I knew that the people I went to work for would find other people to clean for them. […] My pain was all over. I couldn't say where. I couldn't say what made it worse, or even better. […] He [her GP] ended up shouting at me. I know he wasn't angry with me; I could tell he was more angry with himself. But it knocked me back. It wasn't until I found David [her new GP] that I felt someone had really listened.[38]

The stories that we live in shape the way we interpret our healthcare encounter; in turn, this has an impact on our wellbeing. The contextual interpretation of practitioner–patient interaction is the focal point of all medical transactions, and the way that we make meaning from our encounter in that context is central to our flourishing. Again, from a common-sense perspective these finding are logical. The sense of being validated or understood has been shown to affect symptoms such as pain.[39] In the acute model, time is typically a snapshot; a consultation, a test, an injection. But the effectiveness of a treatment is shaped longitudinally by other contexts such as expectations, narratives, the patients' home or work. A typical prescription of a drug is not just about a pharmaceutical, but about a ritual that the patient enacts three times daily until the course of drugs is complete. It is about if their sister reported side effects or success. If they have just been made redundant or are embarking on a new love affair. The patient's interaction with the context for the treatment is characterised by a process of interpretation: a process by which they make their experiences meaningful. As both time and context shift, so does the patient's response. What is clear is that both the Patient and the Doctor need to feel 'safe' during any healthcare interaction, and as far as is possible, have any anxiety alleviated. Both their experiences and understandings of the world need to be validated. This is true of the consultation itself and the wider context of their experience. Context effects are interdependent and, in the case of chronic conditions, experienced over extended time periods and change, therefore to reduce the consultation to isolated elements removed from time and context, is unhelpful. Moreover, when the dominant cultural narrative emphasises the success of the acute model of medicine with its presumed cure, then both are invalidated in their understanding of the world and their roles within it.

Notes

1. As philosopher Roland Barthes suggested, any story or idea that sustains a dominant ideology is naturalised. Barthes, R. *Mythologies* (Paris: Editions du Seuil, 1957).
2. See, for example, Ong, L. M., J. C. De Haes, A. M. Hoos, and F. B. Lammes. "Doctor-Patient Communication: A Review of the Literature." *Social Science & Medicine* 40, no. 7 (1995): 903–918; Kearley, K. E.,

G. K. Freeman, and A. Heath. "An Exploration of the Value of the Personal Doctor-Patient Relationship in General Practice." *British Journal of General Practice* 51, no. 470 (2001): 712–718.
3. Wearne, B. *The Theory and Scholarship of Talcott Parsons to 1951: A Critical Commentary* (Cambridge: Cambridge University Press, 1989).
4. Bennett, Susan. *Theatre Audiences: A Theory of Production and Reception* (Abingdon; New York: Routledge, 1997).
5. Beach, M. C., and T. Inui. "Relationship-Centred Care." *Journal of General Internal Medicine* 21, no. S1 (2006).
6. May, H. *Aristotle's Ethics: Moral Development and Human Nature* (London; New York: Continuum, 2010).
7. Ranheim, A., and H. Dahlberg. "Ecological Caring—Revisiting the Original Ideas of Caring Science." *International Journal of Qualitative Studies on Health and Well-being* 11, no.1 (2016): 33344.
8. www.paintoolkit.org
9. Moore, Pete (1 February 2017) Conversation with Sarah Goldingay, *Royal College of Chiropractors*, Kent Terrace, London.
10. Goldingay, Sarah, P. Dieppe, M. Mangan, and D. Marsden. "(Re)Acting Medicine: Applying Theatre in Order to Develop a Whole-Systems Approach to Understanding the Healing Response." *RiDE Research in Drama Education* 19, no. 3 (2014): 277.
11. Ibid.
12. May, Hope. *Aristotle's Ethics: Moral Development and Human Nature* (London; New York: Continuum, 2010).
13. See www.kingsfund.org.uk "Long-term conditions and multi-morbidity" [Accessed 19/3/17].
14. Le Fanu, J. *The Rise and Fall of Modern Medicine* (New York: Avalon Publishing, 2002); Illich, I. *Medical Nemesis* (London, UK: Calder and Boyars, 1974).
15. Carlson, M. *Performance: A Critical Introduction* (Abingdon, UK: Routledge, 2004); Schechner, R. *Performance Studies: An Introduction*. 3rd ed. (Abingdon, UK: Routledge, 2013); Pitches, J., and S. Popat. *Performance Perspectives: A Critical Introduction* (New York, USA: Palgrave Macmillan, 2011).
16. Goldingay, Sarah. "Contra Mortem, Petimus Scientiam: Pain, Tragedy, Death and Medicine in BLOK/EKO." *Studies in Theatre and Performance* 32, no. 3 (2012): 347–358.
17. Mangan, M. *Staging Ageing: Theatre, Performance and the Narrative of Decline* (Bristol: Intellect, 2013).

18. Schechner, R. *Performance Studies: An Introduction.* 3rd ed. (Abingdon, UK: Routledge, 2013).
19. Schechner, R. *Performance Theory.* Revised ed. (New York, USA; London, UK: Routledge, 1988); Turner, V. *Dramas, Fields and Metaphors* (Ithaca, USA; London, UK: Cornell University Press, 1974).
20. Pavis, P. *Languages of the Stage.* Translated by Susan Melrose, et al. (New York, USA: PAJ Publications, 1982); Alter, J. A. *Sociosemiotic Theory of Theatre* (Philadelphia: University of Pennsylvania Press, 1990).
21. Schechner, R. *Performance Studies: An Introduction.* 3rd ed. (Abingdon, UK: Routledge, 2013).
22. Goldingay, S. "Contra Mortem, Petimus Scientiam: Pain, Tragedy, Death and Medicine in BLOK/EKO." *Studies in Theatre and Performance* 32, no. 3 (2012): 347–358.
23. Franks, A. W. *The Wounded Storyteller: Body, Illness and Ethics* (University of Chicago Press, 2013); Kleinman, A. *The Illness Narratives: Suffering, Healing, and the Human Condition* (Basic Books, 1988); Morris, D. B. *The Culture of Pain* (University of California Press, 1991); wounded storyteller Scarry, E. *The Body in Pain: The Making and Unmaking of the World* (Oxford: Oxford University Press, 1985).
24. Goldingay, S. "Howard Barker." In *Modern British Playwriting: The 80s: Voices, Documents, New Interpretations,* edited by J. Milling (London: Methuen, 2012).
25. Case, G. A. "Performance and the Hidden Curriculum in Medicine." *Performance Research* 19, no. 4 (2014): 6–13.
26. Mangan, M. *The Drama, Theatre and Performance Companion* (Basingstoke: Palgrave, 2013), 125–126.
27. Boal, A. *Theatre of the Oppressed.* Translated by C. and M.-O. Leal McBride (London, UK: Pluto Press, 1979); Freire, P. *Pedagogy of the Oppressed* (London, UK; New York, USA: Continuum, 1970).
28. Becker, H. S., B. Geer, E. C. Hughes, et al. *The Boys in White* (New Brunswick, USA: Transaction Books, 1984).
29. Goldingay, S. (2012–2014). Interviews/Focus Group with First Year Medical Students. Exeter, UK: Unpublished.
30. Mercer, N. *The Guided Construction of Knowledge: Talk Among Teachers and Learners* (Clevedon: Multilingual Matters, 1995).
31. Goldingay, S. (2012–2014). Interviews/Focus Group with First Year Medical Students. Exeter, UK: Unpublished.
32. Goetz, J. L., D. Keltner, E. Simon-Thomas. "Compassion: An Evolutionary Analysis and Empirical Review." *Psychology Bulletin* 136

(2010): 351–374.; Neumann, M., C. Scheffer, D. Tauschel, et al. "Physician Empathy: Definition, Outcome-Relevance and Its Measurement in Patient Care and Medical Education." *GMS Zeitschrift für MedizinischeAusbildung* 29 (2012): Doc11.
33. Jankowiak-Siuda, K., K. Rymarczyk, and A. Grabowska. "How We Empathize with Others: A Neurobiological Perspective." *Medical Science Monitor* 17 (2011): RA18–RA24.
34. Neumann, M., C. Scheffer, D. Tauschel, et al. "Physician Empathy: Definition, Outcome-Relevance and Its Measurement in Patient Care and Medical Education." *GMS Zeitschrift für MedizinischeAusbildung* 29 (2012): Doc11.
35. Goldingay, S., P. Dieppe, M. Farias. "'And the Pain Just Disappeared into Insignificance': The Healing Response in Lourdes—Performance, Psychology and Caring." *The International Review of Psychiatry* 26, no. 3 (2014): 315–323.
36. Rogers, C. R. "The Necessary and Sufficient Conditions of Therapeutic Personality Change." *Journal of Consulting and Clinical Psychology* 60, no. 6 (1992): 827.; Rogers, C. R. *On Becoming a Person* (Boston: Houghton Mifflin, 1961); Watson, J. *Nursing. The Philosophy and Science of Caring* (Boulder: University Press of Colorado, 2008).
37. Osterman, P., and D. Schwartz-Barcott. "Presence: Four Ways of Being There." *Nursing Forum* 31 (1996): 23–30.
38. Goldingay, S. (2016). *Interviews/Fieldnotes*, Blackthorn, Maidstone, Kent. Unpublished.
39. Vangronsveld, D. L., S. J. Linton. "The Effect of Validating and Invalidating Communication on Satisfaction, Pain and Affect in Nurses Suffering from Low Back Pain During a Semi-Structured Interview." *European Journal of Pain* 16 (2012): 239–246.

Sarah Goldingay, PhD, FHEA, FRSA is a senior lecturer in the Department of Drama at the University of Exeter. Trained as an actor, she is a regular contributor to BBC Radio 2 and 4 and a trans-disciplinary scholar whose work has been published in the fields of drama, religion and spirituality, psychiatry and medicine. She explains how the enactment of the clinical encounter is a key factor determining a person's response to any medical intervention and that this encounter is a ritualistic performance.

5

Articulating Pain: Writing the Autoimmune Self

Alice Andrews

Articulations

It hurts. There's kernel of certainty there. It hurts. How to articulate this? Inflammation they say. Swelling they see. Joint disease they diagnose. Pain they presume. I feel a heavy grind, I feel my joints working hard, inefficiently, broken. Friction burns, a resistance that radiates, shrill, smooth and certain. A whiiiine.

'Speaking frightens me because, by never saying enough, I always say too much.'[1] Speaking frightens me and so I begin (again) with the words of another. A quotation of an other, another quotation, where speech becomes constrained, enclosed, within a process of writing that says too little ('who is speaking? And, why should I care?'). It is to this act of writing as a constriction, as an *anguish*—through the narrowing of the *angustia*—that this chapter attends. A certain anguish is, I would suggest, constitutive to the act of writing as it marks the inability to communicate

---

A. Andrews (✉)
Goldsmiths, University of London, London, UK

any experience, to put it into words, to have it understood and responded to. And yet, in addition to the failure of communication, one must attend too to the paradoxical excess of communication that resides within narratives of pain. As words are written, as letters cross the page; as 'scare quotes' signal the scary arrival and departure of others, so that a philosopher's ghost appears through the numeral, an aside to the footnote and all that explodes there in the margins; as the one who says 'I' proliferates as she writes, complains, analyses and argues, ventriloquising all the others that write (with) her pain, be they material, cultural, political or social, human or non-human actors.

This chapter argues that through articulating the paradoxical open closure of the self, particularly through attention to the autobiographical self in pain, one might begin to mark a potential to articulate individualised suffering differently. By beginning from a mode of writing that speaks directly of this experience as a personal experience to which the individual *cannot but attend*, I will suggest that any response to the questions of collective suffering that call for political action needs to attend to the complexities of individualised suffering and attendant self-immunisations through self-care.

The chapter therefore attempts to model a practice of writing the self as a strategy of 'self-care' that is able to locate in the individual a plurivocity of narratives, where the personal, political and theoretical cross to produce different 'worlds' which interconnect in risky and painful ways. Systems theory and Derridean deconstruction perform two alternative ways of thinking of these 'worlds' as 'open closure,' while affect theory touches material bodies, attending to the manner in which feeling is public but also intensely intimate. For, of course, the concern with articulation and writing here is not merely a concern with words alone and a purely discursive present. To 'articulate' is, after all, etymologically connected to the anatomy of joints and limbs: to join, or hinge, bridging a divide between one limb and another, neither one nor the other, inside nor out.[2] Open and closed, joined and separated, the joint marks a site of movement which is necessary for anything to be communicated at all. Both a metaphor and not, these joints translate across limits, marking and inscribing limits between material, psychic, and social worlds. And this movement of the joint can readily become painful.

Bony erosions spreading to joint cartilage. They said they can see it on the x-ray—but I can see nothing. Bone has been grating on bone, I felt it do that, I told them so—they made a mark on a scale, a score out of ten. A particular organisation of atoms, (mis)communications between chemicals and cells, material traces translated via electromagnetic radiation, sensations becoming words, all articulate here as symptoms, and are translated into a diagnosis.

Autoimmunity

The diagnosis in this instance was of autoimmune inflammatory arthritis. The word 'autoimmune' articulating here, alongside the inflamed joints, the linking of a complexity of associations across biomedical, political and philosophical realms. In the movement of the join(t)s between specific autoimmune bodies, one can diagnose, I will suggest, the troubling maintenance of a generalised pain which has become chronic and systemic.

Autoimmune disease refers to a seemingly 'self-inflicted' physiological illness where a body's immune system—which supposedly protects an organism from harm—turns on and against its own constitutive elements, suicidally destroying itself through the very act of defending itself. Autoimmunity names then a paradox at the heart of the modern conception of the bodily self, where 'self' is seen as distinct from an environment conceived as hostile, a self which is obliged to defend itself from such hostility or 'otherness' in order to maintain its self-same ipseity.[3] Self and other, friend and foe, defence and attack are confused in the manifestation of autoimmune disease. And the experience is a painful one.

For one who inherits the legacy of the bioscientific language of immunity, which translates from the juridico-political (immunity-as-exemption) to the militaristic (immunity-as-defence)[4]; for one assured since childhood that threats to bodily integrity are a passing unpleasantness, a temporary hiccup in a life defined by capacity; for one who has come to expect, in respect to the experience of pain, the comfort of a mother or some other; for one assured that the headache will pass on the ingestion of a white pill or two: for this one the diagnosis of autoimmunity and chronic illness is traumatic. A trauma in the expected narrative as calls to 'get well soon!,'

soon cease to be heard. A certain future interrupts the expected present, an elderly decrepitude before one's time; disability and insecurity interrupt the promise of the good life in the moment of an autoimmune crisis.

Repetitive attacks on my joints inscribe my body, wearing down the ligaments, cartilage and bone, in the interval the bone re-grows, locking the joints in place, fusing the gap that allows for movement. Paralysing and petrifying, a certain future is ossified.

But worse. *The urgency of the pain demands a response. I decide to take the immunosuppressant drugs to suppress my over-active immune response, suppressing the bodily self's presumed 'self,' opening my body, again, to the threat of the 'other,' to the hybrid body of the monoclonal human/mouse antibody; to the threat of infections; to the 'side-effects' of the medical-industrial complex. Repeating and confirming the autoimmunity of the immunitary act.*

But worse. Within the logic of autoimmunity there is a crisis of the very concept of self itself marked. The very idea of the *autos*—and thus the autonomy and automaticity that it presumes—comes under attack so that the agency that 'decides' is seen to always already be marked by the other—by the legacy and authority of bioscience and its masters' assumptions, by one's healthcare system, one's autobiography, or the engineered chimeric mouse/human monoclonal antibody that gets under one's skin. A self always already other, and an 'I' always already divided, discernable there in the gap between the 'one' who writes and the 'one' who is written, 'one' always already incapable of deciding autonomously and powerfully for oneself, always already marked violently, painfully, by that which 'one' is not.

But worse, autoimmune reactions proliferate: worse, perhaps, as the solipsistic mourning for this modern Western presumption of an autonomous 'one' obscures the other ones that never knew the comfort of an enveloping care, a medical system, or the assistance of a white pill or two—the ones marked here in the shadow of the (auto)immune 'autos' as 'other.' Ones whose wearing out through the overworking of one's joints comes not as a shock; the 'ones' 'over there' whose symptoms do not translate as diagnoses; the ones whose worn bodies expect nothing different; the ones in the cage, the non-human animals who's pain fails to communicate … one inscribing one another and suffering under the strain of the articulation.

> *In the writing of autoimmune disease autoimmune reactions proliferate and an insecurity is grasped, a motor that drives fear and (auto) immunization.*
>
> But better? As the logic of the *autos* and of immunity translates back from the world of bioscience to that of the juridico-political and the philosophical, can autoimmunity be seen to mark not only a terrifying disease but also a deconstructive promise that might threaten the security of normative narratives of self?

Autoimmunities

Jacques Derrida's appropriation of the bioscientific metaphor of autoimmunity confers on the term a deconstructive force. The term appears with increasing frequency in his late work, where he names biomedical autoimmunity as 'that strange behaviour where a living being, in a quasi-*suicidal* fashion, "itself" works to destroy its own protection, to immunise itself *against* its "own" immunity'[5]; it works, Derrida claims, by 'protecting itself against its self-protection by *destroying its own immune system*.'[6] This seemingly inaccurate (though, perhaps, 'strategic') definition, names autoimmunity as attacking not *any* tissue in the body, but precisely the body's immune system and its ability to defend itself. Thus this definition names the self-opening of a 'body' to whatever or whoever may come.[7]

Finding in all immunitary actions an autoimmunitary reaction every effort to defend 'the self' in Derrida's thinking, forces the inclusion of the other in an autoimmunitary move that *maintains* through (auto)infection. A strange logic then appears where the 'other' in relation to 'self' maintains self—*is* self in that it functions *with* and for the self—even as it reveals the fiction of any stable sense of what 'self' might be.[8] What this autoimmunity produces then is a 'suicide' of the *sui-*, or the *autos* itself, and that this opening to 'whatever comes' is marked as a promise of a survival—figured as *survivance* as *more* life, or *more than* life—a survival of the 'self' through and with the 'other.'[9] Suffering the inscription of the other might, therefore, be figured as the suffering of a certain violent appearance of the other, but one that could mark creative, even joyful, difference. Autoimmunity, after all, marks another iteration of deconstruction itself, supplementing the line of neologisms that Derrida employs: *différance*, the trace, the double-bind, the *pharmakon*, the aporia, and so on.

And yet, in *Rogues*, Derrida figures autoimmunity not as joyful or discomforting, but as painful, even tortuous in the endless revolutions between self-protection (isolation and paralysis) and self-destruction (threat to self-cohesion); Derrida suggests that any 'automobilic and autonomic turn or, rather, return to self, toward the self and upon the self' is a turn upon a torturer's wheel.[10] This automatic re-turn to the power of one 'tortures' in an inquisition 'where one is not only put *in* question but is put *to the* question.'[11] A torturing of the self, by the self that is also a tortuous interrogation by another. Therefore, for Derrida, there appears to be pain and terror on both sides of the autoimmunitary moment. In fact, in the rendition of the deconstructive trace as autoimmunity, deconstruction is nearly always qualified with adjectives such as 'terrifying,' 'terrible,' and 'cruel.'[12] Why this focus on terror in the autoimmunitary lexicon?

Though again better. Again the wheel turns: 'for better *or* worse,' 'in sickness and in health.' The 'law of a terrifying and suicidal autoimmunity,'[13] like the marriage vow, is a contract written in law and maintained in life; it is a mixing of elements, and a joining of worlds. Autoimmune linkages perform for better or worse—for better *and* worse; in sickness *and* in health. And yet the law of autoimmunity, like marriage, risks maintaining normative systems, systems of care and systems of suffering, where some more or less than others become (in)visible under the eyes of its law.

Alarm Bells: Acute Pain

The pain flares. 'Flare up': a term used to describe a sudden and unexpected exacerbation of symptoms. The rumbling inflammation suddenly bursts into flame, bright, urgent, calling for a response. Waking with a pain so violent it makes me tremble: Danger! Phone for an emergency consultation, a new script for the corticosteroids, the 'stress hormone,' fear in a bottle readying one for flight or fight.

But it's difficult to fight when you can't get out of bed. Adapt: I need help to the bathroom; the baby's crying; could you, would you mind…? Let's talk about a system of care: "In sickness and in health?" "No personal independence plan?" "Have you tried…?"

Acute pain is often described as an alarm bell, a warning that the body is in danger: react, move away from the object now perceived as threat and identified as 'bad.'[14] As a communication that instigates an immune response, pain helps to protect an organism from harm. Like the immune system, pain helps a body-as-organism learn appropriate behaviour in relation to one's environment in order to ensure self-maintenance.

Autopoiesis

The painful paradoxes of autoimmunity can be re-articulated within the language of second-order systems theory and its concept of *autopoiesis*.[15] Such a re-articulation speaks to the manner in which acute pain's 'alarm signal' can come to maintain a system of individualised suffering though population-wide chronic pain.

Like autoimmunity, autopoiesis is a term developed in the biosciences, translating the Greek words *autos*—and thus the senses of autonomy and automaticity that attend it—and *poeisis* as the act of making. Against autoimmunity as a deconstructive term and a signifier of a certain self-destruction, we have then autopoiesis as self-creation, and yet in their unfolding these signifying terms become *almost* indistinguishable.

For Humberto Maturana and Francisco Varela—the first to hypothesise autopoiesis in the biosciences—a living system is established upon the distinction between inside and outside, or rather, system and environment.[16] An autopoietic system is a system that can maintain, produce and *creatively* re-produce itself. But it is able to do so only because such a system is founded on a fundamental paradox. An autopoietic system is necessarily both open and closed *at the same time*. The system—and here we could be speaking of any living system, from a cell to an organ to an organism—remains *operationally* closed in regard to its organised function, but *structurally* open to its environment. The result is that in terms of its function an autopoietic system *can know only itself*; it does what it does, repeating and maintaining its own processes self-referentially. Self is self is self for the autopoietic system, anything which lies outside will always remain radically absent to it. However, this tautology forces the system to remain 'structurally coupled' to its environment, entering into any manner of prosthetic relations as it seeks to maintain itself.

Autoimmunity, like the trace, différance, pharmakon, etc. marks within every attempt to maintain, protect, or persist, a spatial and a temporal deferral of pure presence. Autoimmunity, like différance is, in Michael Naas' words, "a deferring of the relationship to the other (whence its immunity [as closure]) and a referral or deference to the other (whence its autoimmunity [as openness])."[17] *Derrida confirms that "[t]his opening is certainly that which liberates time and genesis (even coincides with them), but it is also that which risks enclosing becoming by giving it a form. That which risks stifling force under form."*[18] *Genesis and liberty are closed by an opening that gives it form. This is the condition of possibility of any system according to Derrida. Yet, the stifling of life as poiesis under a certain form does not determine this system, which remains open temporally as well as spatially to a certain excess.*

Environmental changes 'outside' an autopoietic system are noticed by that system operationally only if it perturbs its ability to operate. Known as positive feedback, these perturbations mark in Cary Wolfe's words a 'difference that *makes* a difference.'[19] Perturbations then act as an 'alarm bell' that signals a threat to cohesion and *forces* the system to complicate its structure and modulate its states in an effort to maintain its operation, resulting in a creative evolution of ever more complex systems. A system has no determinate destination, only a tendency to homeostasis, reproducing the code of its organisation, a code that is nonetheless altered on the way under specific historical and material conditions in a creative, adaptive evolution.

Take the immune system, for example.[20] Traditionally conceived, the immune system is housed in a particular organism or 'structure' in order to defend it from the infiltration of the 'other' that may threaten its cohesion. However, from a systems theoretical perspective the immune system 'knows' only itself; it is operationally closed. In also being open to the environment, however, the system is open to the other. Yet, any 'other' that comes 'within' and which does not perturb the systemic operation is

5 Articulating Pain: Writing the Autoimmune Self 91

not reacted to—its status as either other or self becomes undecidable. If the alarm bell is rung, the immune system will react. The bioscientist Polly Matzinger proposes, following a similar logic, a 'danger model' of the immune system, where the immune system is seen to respond not to 'foreignness' but to local events that signal 'danger'; it is the quantitative disturbance *within* the organism that causes a reaction.[21]

So too for Derrida. A system knows only itself: "every other is wholly other"[22] *even while it bears the trace of the other. And yet, a difference is marked. For Derrida, the distinction between positive feedback as a difference that makes a difference and negative feedback as a difference that maintains the same operation, is less clearly defined. A perturbation that maintains a system and is therefore not 'noticed' by it (the food we eat, the non-threatening bacteria), and the perturbation that rings the alarm bell necessitating that an adaptation or compensation be made, both appear to fundamentally disturb, as, for Derrida, every 'perturbation' in some sense marks a certain violence:*

> *As soon as there is the One, there is murder, wounding, traumatism.* L'Un se garde de l'autre. *The One guards against/keeps some of the other. It protects itself from the other, but, in the movement of this jealous violence, it comprises in itself, thus guarding it, the self-otherness or self-difference (the difference from within oneself) which makes it One. The "One differing, deferring from itself." The One as the Other. At once, at the same time, but in a time that is out of joint, the One forgets to remember itself to itself, it keeps and erases the archive of injustice that it is. Of this violence that it does.* L'Un se fait violence.[23]

The 'violence' that Derrida speaks of here is clearly disturbing, it is 'murder, wounding, traumatism,' and it is not a *particular* 'other' that disturbs, but 'otherness.' This other is *necessarily* violent. A suffering of the other by the one. In part this violence could be seen as the violence of material inscriptions as systems force differences on one another, but, for Derrida, it is also the violence of the foundational paradox, or aporia, which unravels logic and the inherited western system that produces and maintains a metaphysics of presence, or what Derrida calls logocentricism.[24] A logocentricism which is productive of the assumptions of power and autonomy of self in modern immunology that render autoimmune pain so traumatising for its individualised subjects. However, what systems theory indicates—employing a very similar reasoning—is that this contradiction, this violence against reason, is just as likely to maintain a system as it is to deconstruct it, in fact one might insist that it is *more* likely to do so.

In *Social Systems*[25] Niklas Luhmann extends the scope of Maturana and Varela's biological autopoiesis to a general field of enquiry that includes psychic and social systems.[26] For Luhmann, the paradox of self-referentiality, and the resulting undecidability between self and other as the foundation of any system is, as it is for Derrida, read as a threat to the unity and closure of the system. However, Luhmann characterises such contradictions not as points from which to begin deconstructing the system, but as the 'alarm bell' of the social system's immune system, which provokes the social system to maintain itself through a structural coupling to other autopoietic systems.

Within a system one is confined within the tautology of self-referentiality. However, stepping *outside* the system provides a site from which one is able to make observations and therefore view a system as being structurally coupled to other autopoietic unities where the distinction between self and other can be reorganised and maintained.[27] So that, in Maturana and Varela's words, 'we can see a unity in *different* domains depending on the distinctions we make.'[28] It is from the position of the observer 'outside' of these domains that these unities and differences are correlated and from where one is able to narrate the co-implication of a system's processes to maintain a 'knowledge' of that system's functions.

The act of writing the self puts one outside oneself, rendering discernable a self as a bounded being (a body as an organism, a consciousness) and its openness to the prosthetic other, a prosthetic 'I': "who is the subject of this utterance, ever alien to the subject of its statement whose intruder it certainly is [...].'[29]

A social system employing meaning as communication, or a psychic system employing meaning as consciousness can observe and maintain the inter-dependence and distinction of self and other in any one system, making them signify in the operation of ever more complex social systems. At each stage of observation however, a new founding distinction is made between system and environment and an increasingly complex environment is coupled to the *operation* of the observation and *its* autopoietic closure *which remains constitutively 'blind' to its other.*

5 Articulating Pain: Writing the Autoimmune Self   93

I feel the arthritic joints that limit my mobility as my autoimmune body's self-referentiality impacts my physiological, not to mention my social, life. It is from this position of this 'I' that can say 'my' that a system of meaning is produced to give me form. Meaning production allows for the coupling of this psychic system to the communications of the medical system that enables me to say "I have autoimmune inflammatory arthritis." It is the coupling of this medical system to the political economy of neoliberal 'care' and 'austerity measures' of the UK in 2016, that determines which bodies are treated and which are not. It is the coupling of this medical system, and this psychic system, with the contingencies of history and its immunological metaphors that risks turning injuries into a war between 'them and us.' But within this increasingly complex set of embedded systems it remains that each system remains constitutively 'blind' to that which it is not, and that which it cannot see (coming).

The paradox of alterity cannot be dispelled; it is merely shifted and must reappear in the new autopoietic social system that protects it. It is, therefore, the constant requirement of psychic and social systems to shift and render harmless the contradictions that threaten their continued survival, responding to the 'alarm signal' of painful perturbations. As Gunter Teubner suggests in his comparative analysis of Derrida and Luhmann:

> Paradoxes not only threaten the structures of social systems [...], against which they must defend, separate and protect themselves; more importantly, paradoxes provoke [systems] into the relentless production of new rules and routines. The actual deconstructive obsession is not with defensive, conservative systems maintaining their original structures but with their insatiable impulse for the invention of new differences. The birth of autopoiesis from the spirit of deconstruction?[30]

Derrida insists: every difference makes a difference, there is disturbance—or 'pain'—in every possible mark, and this pain deconstructs every unity. Systems theory insists: violence can be tolerated, and where it cannot the system will adapt or die. Both insist: this is a description of what happens and not a prescription.[31] Deconstruction or reconstruction? For both the decision is undecidable. And yet the decision is made. Yet, in a social and political environment where the powerful 'system' of logocentricism has been inherited, where narratives that fear pain and invest in the search for pleasure are reproduced and circulated, the *chance* inherent in both systems theory and deconstruction's openness to the event appear as frozen promises, and deconstruction's paradoxes facilitate the *re*construction of powerful political norms. This is a 'reconstruction' that *maintains* pain not as a perpetual violence that makes a difference, but as chronic pain not only managed but also maintained and produced as a necessary component of the functioning of a socio-political system of (neo)liberal governance. How might an individualised self-enmeshed within these intersecting worlds, worn out, pained and incapacitated in multiple ways, ever begin to write these narratives differently?

Alarm Bells: Chronic Pain

The genetic marker HLA-B27 writes letters in my blood. From father to daughter a genetic legacy is passed, yet its message is received differently. There was no effective treatment before the arrival of the bioengineered antibodies and so for the father: chronic pain, isolating and boring, insistent and dull, the alarm bell rings in silence, a tinnitus that makes one deaf to others. Slowly the articulation of his joints failed, a frozen chance determined by the articulations of genetic, medical, social, political limits, all locked within an increasingly rigid socio-political encoding of pain as disability, as suffering and insufferable, isolating and petrifying.

Despite the essential indeterminacy of all systems in their creative autopoietic adaptation, a certain effect of sovereign power appears as the 'reason of the strongest' wins out,[32] and, as Joseph Vogl suggests, despite the proliferation of difference within the prosthetic articulations of the 'human' and 'posthuman,' a particular form of 'man' as *homo economicus* has succeeded to maintain himself in multiple fields,[33] and despite the abundance of novel formulations, a particular form of liberal governance persists through its intimate coupling with multiple systems, including the social, political, medical and cultural.

Vogl suggests that *homo economicus* has endured since the end of the Middle Ages because he is concerned not with determining truth or falsity, the just or the unjust, but only with maintaining profit and loss through adaptability and readiness to reform. Thus

5 Articulating Pain: Writing the Autoimmune Self 95

[*homo economicus*] can be understood as a medium that produces economic as well as social systems. When we speak of a 'poetics of homo economicus', we mean to investigate this human type from the perspective of his fabrication, his *poiesis*; to grasp him as both a subject and object of cultural practices.[34]

This *poiesis* of the human form that produces economic as well as social systems would be *auto*poietic in Luhmann's account,[35] a form as an operation that functions through a self-affirmation—or self-interest—but which necessitates interaction with others in what systems theory would call a structural coupling. For *homo economicus*, simple self-interest that directs the individual 'towards pleasure and away from pain' (that is, away from risky perturbation and towards a creative homeostasis) leads that individual to manage risk through calculation, insurance, and interest, sustaining in the process more complex systems of economic and social support structures—sustaining, that is, productivity and economic value within a free market. As a complex autopoietic system the individual remains necessarily oblivious to the complexity of his environment. This individual maintains himself by turning what Vogl calls a 'blind eye' to the complex inscriptions of the 'other' in an effort to envisage his desire: a promise of the good life free from pain.

Turning away from pain, turning towards pleasure, with each turn of the screw, tortuous autoimmunity marks itself again for this liberal individual. The promise of pleasure is cruel; it arrives only in the form of pain and is maintained by cultural and personal narratives that articulate the individual. Since the nineteenth century and the machinations of industry—if not before—the desire for pleasure and the individual's relation to future abundance, as what Lauren Berlant figures as the 'good life,' comes to be sustained only through the cruelty of wear and tear, fatigue and exhaustion of the present.[36] Work harder today for greater rewards tomorrow—a promise as a salve that marks an autoimmune suffering. As the creative adaptability of the liberal system wins out and as liberalism becomes neoliberalism, the operation of the free market and its laws are no longer a subsystem of society *alongside* those of politics, law, art, and so on. but *its operation is extended over them*. From the perspective of the overarching neoliberal system then, Vogl suggests, *homo economicus* becomes both an abstraction, de-individualised as an example or a statistic, *and* an individualised resource as her everyday life, hopes, dreams—and aches and pains—are mined for their future economic value; while the autopoietic individual in crisis *within* this injurious system remains 'blind' to this complexity.[37]

As Lauren Berlant insists, the particular 'crises' produced by the labouring body under neoliberal capitalism are crises in name only. The 'obesity crisis' or 'chronic pain crisis' does not perform as a crisis, for if a crisis marks a decisive point, a moment of danger and risk that necessitates a decision, then the 'ordinary crisis' of failing bodies provokes no decision, and no moment of danger that perturbs the system that produces it[38] Such 'events' or 'crises' are narrated as crises in the media and scientific literature, Berlant suggests, without *performing* as crises.[39] The rhetoric of 'crisis' belies the fact that such sufferings are structural and ubiquitous: the suffering experienced and the language used to communicate this in the terminology of systems theory, produces differences and, perturbed by this violence, the system adapts—as liberal capitalism is so ready to do. But there is no difference marked here *that makes a difference to the operation of the system that maintains this suffering*. Nothing here threatens to imperil the sovereign system which therefore does not—or cannot—respond responsibly to the suffering it facilitates.

Such systems adapt to the painful perturbations of its operation by *incorporating* pain and suffering into the profitability of the system as chronic pain. Chronic pain here then, I would suggest, is a pain that not only persists but which is also maintained beyond its usefulness as an alarm and a signal for action. In chronic pain the alarm continues to ring, deafening one to the possibility of a different present or future not necessarily structured by the cruel optimisms of a promised cure.

HLA B27 inscribes itself differently as an acute and insistent pain comes to refer this 'one' to 'advances' in the pharmaceutical industry. Inflammation and erosions signal less a certain disability, and more a symptom that maps a treatment plan: a drug regime, a diet, pain management techniques and stress reduction strategies. 'Have you tried the new biosimilars?' 'Did you hear about the new bioelectronics?' 'Have you tried massage? Mindfulness? Yoga? …' Pain managed in this way comes to refer less to disability than to what Jaspir Puar calls 'debility' as a certain weakness.[40] *A rendition of pain that weakens but which—by entering into an economy of care of the medical and 'wellbeing' industries, deeply invested in the discourses of cure and the logic of maintenance—does not render one unfit for work.*

The medical-industrial complex's investment in curing disability and healing suffering invests in the assumption that pain is to be avoided at all costs; this makes it difficult, as Alyson Patsavas argues, to code pain as anything other than tragic—so overvaluing the promise of a cure.[41] However, the medical-industrial complex's investment in curing disability functions in tandem with pressures to work longer hours which maintains pain and the demand for its cure. And further, as Jaspir Puar has forcefully argued, the binary of disabled/nondisabled can be deconstructed; it becomes less a case of distinguishing between who is disabled and who is not—but through what Puar calls the 'accommodation of degrees'—to what *degree* is one disabled, and what might the appropriate treatment be?[42] Perhaps a glass of wine at the end of a hard day? Or a daily drug regime, as bodies and populations enter into the interacting autopoietic systems of the medical-industrial complex, health insurance, or state benefits. Each pain, and each response providing a feedback loop that maintains the profitability of debility, as population-wide chronic pain.

Testimony

> *Last night at school I walked across the street to the parking garage and climbed six floors to the top. I walked to the edge and stood on the railing thinking about how I would rather not live than be in pain all my life. I don't know how long I stood there, but in the moment I fully rationalized dying. Death is full of happiness, exemption from this suffering.*[43]

This, Alyson Patsavas' powerful personal account of her reaction to a diagnosis of chronic pain is taken from her pain journals and quoted in her article 'Recovering a Cripistemology of Pain.' This quotation offers an account of the traumatic effects of a diagnosis of chronic pain that has been culturally determined as insufferable. Patsavas tactically employs her pain and her trauma in what she terms a 'cripistemology' which combines knowledge produced through a specific autobiographical standpoint and a process of 'cripping' which 'spins mainstream representations or practices to reveal able-bodied assumptions.'[44] This strategy of writing the self in relation to complex systems attempts to mark a difference that makes a difference within the autopoietic self-maintenance of the culture industries, industries which maintain themselves through the *flexible* reproduction of narratives of inclusion, care and cure, which comes to directly affect systemic forms of suffering.[45] We could think here, for example, of the 2016 film *Me Before You*[46] which presents chronic pain as insufferable, or the advertisements in the UK labelling Paralympians as 'superhuman' reducing them to a mere cultural memes for the inspiration of the able-bodied to work harder to achieve their 'good lives,' or the repeated accounts of chronic pain sufferers as drug addicts in the TV show *House M.D.* contributing to prescription laws that drastically limit access to pain relief.[47]

Patsavas' testimony seeks in part to challenge such normative narratives by bearing witness to a personal suffering through an act of writing that is able to observe the paradoxes of the individualised body and see these as coupled to broader socio-cultural ableist logic in order to begin to deconstruct both, but it also provides a platform for marginalised identities to render their embodied existences readable across social divides. Pain narratives provide a powerful means for collectivising marginalised identities, for as Sara Ahmed suggests, despite pain's essential incommunicability pain provokes translation and communication, and comes to be constantly evoked in public discourse as that which 'demands a collective as well as individual response.'[48]

Patasvas' response attempts to recover collective responsibility from within the structural limitations of the individual. However, often, as Lauren Berlant warns, the use of personal pain in public discourse becomes problematic. In the movement from the personal to the collective there is a risk of collective *over*-identification with pain so that one risks becoming *passive* to the experience as a marker of one's identity, turning a 'blind eye' to the complex inscriptions of the other; and further, the 'truth value' that individualised narratives of pain come to embody, in addition to making them potent tools in calls for social justice, also threatens to obscure *structural* sufferings.[49]

5 Articulating Pain: Writing the Autoimmune Self 99

Berlant suggests that the assumption that sharing stories of suffering provides a map for achieving the good life if only we would cure the suffering assumes that these accounts of pain can be acutely felt by the social and political systems it attempts to disrupt. It assumes that such accounts have a power to perturb these systems. However, in subscribing to the logic of the cure and attempting to treat the pain of the other in a pursuit of communal happiness, such strategies contribute to narratives of pain avoidance and pleasure seeking through promising pleasure and achieving pain that enter into an economy of return. For, as both Ahmed and Berlant remark, the only pain that really comes to matter in many calls for social justice is the pain that makes the one that attempts to *treat* it feel better.[50]

Therefore, rather than a model of trauma (or what I have been calling 'acute pain') which sustains a faith in the emergency response and amelioration through protective immunitary systems, Berlant calls for a model of suffering. For, she claims, 'suffering' speaks etymologically of pain and patience, and would present not singular acts of violence that can be confronted and remedied, but rather a generalised atmosphere of violence (or what I have been calling chronic pain). Berlant goes on, however in parentheses, to trouble her use of the term 'suffering':

> But even *suffering* can sound too dramatic for the subordinated personhood form I am reaching toward here: imagine a word that describes a constantly destabilised existence that monitors, with a roving third eye, every moment as a potentially bad event in which a stereotyped one might become food for someone else's hunger for superiority and connect that to a term that considers the subjective effects of structural inequalities that are deemed inevitable in a capitalist nation. *Suffering* stands in for that compound word.[51]

I can imagine a compound word that speaks of a constantly destabilised existence, where every event is potentially bad, a word that connects to subjective effects of structural inequalities. Here *autoimmunity* stands in for that compound word.

Time Is Out of Joint

Autoimmunity returns us to the *autos* as a self that can know only itself, that is individual, specific, personal, and isolated *at the same time* as it is maintained in a prosthetic relation to others that renders this individuality impossible, painfully deconstructing it. Like autopoiesis, like chronic pain, deconstructive autoimmunity enacts a protection which is painful and violent, where all immunity is an opening to the other, another which is at once self *and* other, an articulation between different worlds. This other within the self is marked as a violence, the anguish of an inscription that is in a certain sense chronic in that it persists. However, in autoimmunity this violence is not figured as that which comes to maintain a central operation, but as that which retains the potential to disrupt. This subtle but significant difference in these theories of survival—autopoiesis or autoimmunity—arises in this historical context due to the differing relation to 'the future' and to 'difference,' and what these words might come to articulate.

I have attempted to suggest that systems which privilege maintenance—as self-interest and an orientation towards pleasure and away from pain—have emerged in this story as powerful systems out of the conditions of Western modernity. One increasingly powerful system has come to be known as neoliberalism, a system that thrives on adaptability, individualises pain, and maintains an operation that invests in the value of future value. And this system, so practised at adapting to forms of resistance, fashions a present in which it is increasingly difficult for other futures to become imaginable.[52] The present is haunted by this inheritance and this promise.

From a specific site of individualised suffering within Western discourses of chronic pain the demand to attend, treat, and respond to one's pain through 'structural couplings' to the medical-industrial complex and optimistic cultural narratives becomes increasingly difficult to resist, or even testify to, as one is continually forced to maintain oneself as a *productive* member of society. Personal narratives and 'cripistemologies' such as Patsavas' respond to this and begin to suggest a mode of writing from specific conditions that might also begin to destabilise these conditions, yet such writings also risk autoimmunely entering into a politics of over-identification with suffering that could render the subjective form passive. Yet, in the practice of writing, in the spaces that appear between the 'I' that is written and the 'I' that writes, in the frightening constriction of the 'I' that speaks, autoimmune openings appear. So, while Berlant speaks of suffering, and cruel optimism, I prefer to speak autoimmunely, where individuals' defence mechanisms are seen to always turn on and against them, opening to the unexpected. Cruel optimism is a panacea, it works despite its cruelty; but autoimmunity is *terrifying*, a terror that catches one's breath, disabling one's ability to participate in the logic of the cure, and of any certain future.

Autoimmunity is always *terrifying* for it acknowledges that one is always running into danger without being prepared for it. Where systems theory focuses on the fact that an operation is maintained until it is not—that is, it is always positioned *within the system* and its paradoxical relation to its 'outside' is ignored—Derrida's autoimmunity attends to the fact that each and every system is always in relation to that which it cannot relate to—to the radically unknowable other outside whose difference makes a difference—to the radically unforeseeable future that arrives unexpectedly. That is, deconstruction's 'roving eye' is always positioned *within the paradox* of an unrelenting, unrelating relation: an articulation with a past and a future which is always out of joint.

In a deconstructive 'system' the only thing that is actively maintained is this paradox, meaning that this future when it arrives is *always* traumatising. For Derrida the trauma cannot be overcome for it is a trauma that hasn't happened yet; it comes as the 'future to come' (*à venir*), which 'can only be anticipated in the form of an absolute danger. It is that which breaks absolutely with constituted normality.'[53] And 'efforts to attenuate or neutralize the effect of the traumatism (to deny, repress, or forget it, to get over it) are but so many desperate attempts. And so many autoimmunitary movements.'[54]

Does the writing of a pained self maintain or deconstruct individualised systems of oppression? An autoimmune writing could not, of course, predict this. Yet it is here in the writing of a self—which cannot (but) communicate a pain that says too little and too much—that the trauma of the future can be felt and maintained, and thus so too the chance to write pained bodies differently, conceiving of a life lived not as immunitary survival through identitarian politics but autoimmune *sur-vivance* that is *more* life and *more* than life, a life crossed with a multiplicity of others. De-individualising gestures, however, do not happen in the abstract; they open onto specific moments of on-going violence and a plurality of worlds and must speak to others from there—saying both too little and too much. For the articulation of the joints *hurt* and they demand my attention.

Notes

1. Derrida, Jacques. *Writing and Difference*. Translated by Alan Bass (London: Routledge and Kegan Paul, 1978), 9. In saying too little of Derrida's writing here, I let his work on the margin do its work from the margins throughout.
2. For a discussion of the etymology of 'articulation' in Derrida's work see: Johnson, Christopher. *System and Writing in the Philosophy of Jacques Derrida* (Cambridge: Cambridge University Press, 1993), 153.
3. Burnet, F. M. *Self and Notself: Cellular Immunology, Book one* (Carlton, VIC and London: Melbourne University Press and Cambridge University Press, 1969).
4. For an account of the history of immunity see: Cohen, Ed. *A Body Worth Defending: Immunity, Biopolitics, and the Apotheosis of the Modern Body* (Durham, NC: Duke University Press, 2009).
5. Derrida, Jacques, and Giovanna Borradori. "Autoimmunity: Real and Symbolic Suicides—A Dialogue with Jacques Derrida." In *Philosophy in a Time of Terror* (Chicago: University of Chicago Press, 2003), 94.
6. Derrida, Jacques. "Faith and Knowledge: The Two Sources of 'Religion' at the Limits of Reason Alone." In *Religion: Cultural Memory in the Present*, edited by J. Derrida and G. Vattimo (Stanford, CA: Stanford University Press, 1988), 73 n. 27, my emphasis.
7. Here Derrida seems to be taking AIDS as a model, for it is in AIDS that the immune system itself is attacked. However, AIDS is not considered an autoimmune disease as the 'attack' is the result of a viral infection and not the body's defensive actions. The apparent error in Derrida's definition of autoimmunity in light of the dominant medical definition, could, however, be reframed as accurate given alternative models of the immune system.

8. This autoimmune logic is not confined, of course, to any particular subjectivity capable of knowing itself but all bodies or all forms organised as self-maintenance.
9. See Derrida, Jacques. "Living On." In *Deconstruction and Criticism*, edited by H. Bloom (New York: The Seabury Press, 1979), 62–141.
10. Derrida, Jacques. *Rogues*. Translated by P.-A. Brault and M. Naas (Stanford, CA: Stanford University Press, 2005), 10.
11. Ibid., 7.
12. For example, in 'Faith and Knowledge' 'this terrifying but inescapable logic of the autoimmunity of the unscathed' (1998, 73), and in *Rogues*: 'the law of a terrifying and suicidal autoimmunity' (2005, 18). Derrida's discussions of autoimmunity circle around the politics of terror, sovereignty, and democracy.
13. Ibid., 18.
14. Doley, Daniel M. *Pain: Dynamics and Complexities* (Oxford; New York: Oxford University Press, 2014), 171.
15. See Johnson, *System and Writing* and Wolfe, Cary. *What Is Posthumanism?* (Minneapolis, MN: University of Minnesota Press, 2010) for important analyses of the relations between deconstruction and systems theory.
16. Maturana, Humberto R., and Francisco J. Varela. *Autopoiesis and Cognition: The Realization of the Living* (Dordrecht; London: Reidel, 1980).
17. Nass, Michael. *Derrida from Now On* (Fordham University Press, 2008), 135.
18. Derrida, *Writing and Difference*, 26.
19. Wolfe, *Posthumanism*, 18.
20. For a discussion of the immune system as autopoietic see: Varela, Francisco J., and Mark R. Anspach. "The Body Thinks: The Immune System and the Process of Somatic Individuation." In *Materialities of Communication*, edited by H. U. Gumbrecht and K. L. Pfeiffer (Stanford, CA: Stanford University Press, 1994), 273–285.
21. Matzinger, Polly. "The Danger Model: A Renewed Sense of Self." *Science* 296 (2002): 301–305. See also Pradeu, Thomas. *The Limits of the Self: Immunology and Biological Identity*. Translated by Elizabeth Vitanza (Oxford: Oxford University Press, 2012).
22. Derrida, Jacques. *The Gift of Death*. Translated by David Wills (Chicago: University of Chicago Press, 1995), 84.

23. Derrida, Jacques. *Archive Fever: A Freudian Impression*. Translated by E. Prenowitz (Chicago: University of Chicago Press, 1996), 78.
24. Derrida, Jacques. *Of Grammatology*. Translated by G. C. Spivak (Baltimore; London: Johns Hopkins University Press, 1976).
25. Luhmann, Niklas. *Social Systems* (Stanford, CA: Stanford University Press, 1995).
26. While the autopoiesis of an organism is secured by form maintaining 'life,' in social systems what is secured is the connective capacity of actions (Luhmann, *Social Systems*, 372).
27. The ocular metaphors of 'observation' and 'blind spots' are repeated throughout the language of systems theory, this language risks both an ableist privileging sight and the introduction of assumptions of knowledge and power that attends metaphors of vision. I continue to use this language here for clarity's sake, yet the meaning should be understood more in regards to capacities to attend.
28. Maturana, Humberto R., and Francisco J. Varela. *The Tree of Knowledge: The Biological Roots of Human Understanding* (Boston: Shambhala, 1987), 135.
29. Nancy, Jean-Luc. 'The Intruder.' In *Corpus* (New York: Fordham University Press, 2008), 162.
30. Teubner, Gunther. "Economics of Gift—Positivity of Justice: The Mutual Paranoia of Jacques Derrida and Niklas Luhmann." *Theory Culture Society* 18, no. 29 (2001): 39.
31. Luhmann, *Social Systems*, 83.
32. This logic of the reason of the strongest is described by Derrida throughout *The Beast and the Sovereign*.
33. I employ the masculine gender here in order associate the *autos* of the modern individual with the Latin *ipse* as "he himself," and the Sovereign of western modernity. See Derrida, *Rogues*, 12.
34. Vogl, Joseph. "Poetics of Homo Economicus." *Continent* 4, no. 1 (2014): 95.
35. Luhmann, Niklas. "The Individuality of the Individual: Historical Meanings and Contemporary Problems." In *Reconstructing Individualism: Autonomy, Individuality, and the Self in Western Thought*, edited by Thomas C. Heller, et al. (Stanford, CA: Stanford University Press, 1986).
36. Berlant, Lauren. *Cruel Optimism* (Durham, NC: Duke University Press, 2011).
37. This marks the diffusion of the power where the reason of the strongest no longer rests with a sovereign individual but perhaps a 'sovereign' *sys-*

tem of neoliberal governance, which Michel Foucault calls in *The Birth of Biopolitics* and elsewhere, 'governmentality.'
38. Berlant, Lauren. "Slow Death (Sovereignty, Obesity, Lateral Agency)." *Critical Inquiry* 33, no. 4 (2007): 754–780.
39. Berlant, "Slow Death," 760.
40. Puar, Jaspir. "The Cost of Getting Better: Suicide, Sensation, Switchpoints." *GLQ* 18, no. 1 (2011): 149–158.
41. Patsavas, Alyson. "Recovering a Cripistemology of Pain: Leaky Bodies, Connective Tissue, and Feeling Discourse." *Journal of Literary & Cultural Disability Studies* 8, no. 2 (2014): 208.
42. Puar, "The Cost of Getting Better," 156.
43. Patsavas, "Recovering a Cripistemology of Pain," 204.
44. Carrie Sandahl quoted in ibid., 205.
45. See McRuer, Robert. *Crip Theory: Cultural Signs of Queerness and Disability* (New York: New York University Press, 2006), 18.
46. Sharrock, Thea, dir. *Me Before You* (Warner Bros. Pictures, 2016).
47. Shore, David, writer. *House M.D.* (Universal Studios Home Entertainment, 2005).
48. Ahmed. "The Contingency of Pain." In *The Cultural Politics of Emotion* (Edinburg: Edinburgh University Press, 2014), 20–41, 20.
49. Berlant, Lauren. "The Subject of True Feeling: Pain, Privacy, and Politics." In *Cultural Pluralism, Identity Politics, and the Law*, edited by Austin Sarat and Thomas R. Kearns (Ann Arbor: The University of Michigan Press, 1999).
50. Ahmed, "The Contingency of Pain," 20.
51. Berlant, "The Subject of True Feeling," 78–79.
52. Mark Fisher. *Ghosts of My Life: Writings on Depression, Hauntology and Lost Futures* (London: Zero Books, 2014).
53. Derrida and Borradori, "Autoimmunity," 99.
54. Ibid.

Alice Andrews is a lecturer in Visual Cultures in the Department of Visual Cultures, Goldsmiths, University of London. Her research is concerned with practices of care in regard to the intersections between medical, philosophical, personal, and political articulations of health and illness. She has a particular interest in the employment of the logic of immunity and autoimmunity in Jacques Derrida's late work.

6

Exhibiting Pain, Death and Grief: From the Art Gallery to the Image Shared Online

Montse Morcate

Pain, death and grief have always been very delicate photographic subjects, not only in documentary or journalistic photography but also and most especially in contemporary art. While photographs portraying grief and death were once an intrinsic part of the family album, these were progressively put away from view, leaving an important lack of visual references of what common pain and grief look like and contributing to their ostracism. As a response, many artists have felt the need to explore their ability to express their visions of suffering and mortality through their cameras, even when this meant crossing the boundaries of what others considered appropriate to photograph or exhibit. In this sense there are two major approaches to these subjects, which I refer to here as the detached approach versus the self-referential approach. For the analysis of this type of works, it matters whether the artist is involved in the story he or she portrays. This involvement affects not only the reaction of the viewer but also the exposure that the

M. Morcate (✉)
University of Barcelona, Barcelona, Spain

© The Author(s) 2018
EJ Gonzalez-Polledo, J. Tarr (eds.), *Painscapes*,
https://doi.org/10.1057/978-1-349-95272-4_6

work receives. Sometimes, these projects have had difficulty reaching the galleries or have received negative reviews; on other occasions, artists have been publicly rebuked or had their work censored by galleries and museums who deemed it offensive to the viewer, or simply not profitable.

Beyond art criticism, art projects dealing with pain, grief or death have an intrinsic value and power that exceeds art itself insofar as they make everyday pain visible for many people in a world where images of suffering and death seem to be reserved for "newsworthy material." Because of the clear capacity of the camera to serve as a mediator of pain and grief, in recent decades photographic projects dealing with these issues have gradually become a very powerful instrument for normalising the grief process of the artist, through the publication of self-referential images of pain, grief and death as part of art projects in exhibitions, catalogues and photo books.

Now, at the turn of the new century, digital images and the Internet have made pain and grief within the family and in intimate territories increasingly visible. In this context, artists now have the opportunity to share their images online not only as ordinary social media users communicating their feelings and experiences of facing pain, death and grief but also, and especially, as artists who can overcome the limitations of the art market by sharing their images online. By doing so, artists can now reach potentially unlimited audiences, receive immediate and continuous feedback from their followers, bring people with common experiences together (helping to build communities of peers) and also offer a new imagery to which other people in grief or pain might relate.

By analysing art works that tackle the subjects of pain and grief and their reception in the context of the art world, especially their impact when shared online, this chapter aims to examine the photo art project's role as a mediator of the artist's grief, its impact on the audience and its value as something that increases visibility and raises awareness of the issues of illness and death by being shared online.

Pain, Death and Grief Photographed: The Detached Versus the Self-referential Approach

Photographic representations of pain, grief and death have been present in important ways since the invention of the medium, as evidenced by the literature on the different forms of photography in the nineteenth century, which produced the earliest representations of death and grief in the family circle.[1] The photographic camera has proved to be an important ally for documenting society's private rites of passage such as weddings and births, but also funerals and deaths. The fact that many of the latter images were once proudly preserved in family albums and even hung on the parlour walls in many Western homes indicates how important it was for people to share those experiences with relatives and acquaintances. The diverse prints they left behind of mourning portraits shared as mementos or sent abroad to the relatives who could not attend a funeral reflected the need of the bereaved to make their loss real and visible by communicating it through photography. At the same time, an analysis of grieving images,[2] including the numerous portraits commissioned by parents who would pose for the camera with their deceased loved one (so creating an allegorical image of pain and grief), reveals that these photographs served not only to capture the likeness of the deceased for posterity's sake but also to ensure that the parents were acknowledged as the bereaved.

Although those early photographic practices were developed and socially accepted during the twentieth century, they gradually declined owing to their perceived inappropriateness in a world where images of mourning and death were considered blemishes on the family photo album, itself the ultimate idealised portrayal of the happy family's visual memory.

Under these new circumstances, the representation of everyday pain and grief was locked behind closed doors and the practice of capturing those moments with the camera became a private and often shameful activity that never ceased but was undertaken secretly and silently. Many photographs of this kind were thrown away, burnt or otherwise destroyed, while others were kept hidden for years as treasured but secret family possessions. During the twentieth century, especially in many Western countries, the changes in the way people accepted and perceived the values of photographic representations of death and grief were inevitably determined by transformations in society's attitudes towards pain, illness, grief and death.[3] First, society had to face a long and turbulent period of war that forced people to bury what gradually became a permanent and depressing condition of mourning. In addition, unprecedented developments in medicine put the onus on human beings to challenge and defeat illness, suffering and ultimately death, pushing the ordinariness of death ever further away.

And yet in spite of this, in the last third of the twentieth century the desert where private and personal suffering had found nothing but drought slowly began to bloom with photographic art projects dealing with grief, pain and death. First, these came as a response to the dearth of images showing ordinary people's pain and grief as opposed to the increasing exposure of images of the suffering of "the other" (perceived by the viewer as geographically, socially and emotionally remote) by the mass media.[4] Second, cancer and HIV/AIDS, two of the most serious and widely feared illnesses in Western countries, threatened to topple the common belief that at least in the richest and allegedly most developed areas of the world medicine could defeat illness and, consequently, death.

In short, towards the end of the last century many artists began to see photography as an appropriate medium for exploring their personal visions of life and death, which in many cases stemmed from their own personal stories and the illness and grief that they or those in their intimate circle had experienced.

In order to understand artists' reasons for addressing such delicate issues and the nature of the art projects they undertake, it is important to distinguish between works that explore illness or death as a general subject from which the artist remains detached, and self-referential projects that aim to explore and narrate a personal experience as a result of grief.[5]

The first group tends to include the works which generate greater controversy among the public and more often receive negative reviews. Some of the artists in this group take the subject of the human corpse to offer their reflections on death, like Jeffrey Silverthorne in his controversial *The Morgue Series* (1972–1974) or Andrés Serrano in *The Morgue* (1992), which both present pictures of people who died from very different causes, ranging from illnesses and accidents of different kinds to murder. Although their visual approach and attitude towards death differ, both give shape to their portrayal of death in the form of the dead stretched out in the transient setting of a morgue: in the form of cadavers that are anonymous—although also totally recognisable as individuals in the case of Silverthorne. These become the object of the camera's scrutiny, an effect which in Serrano's work is enhanced by the use of the large-format camera, and they mirror the uncertain destiny that our own loved ones and even we ourselves must be ready for. But the fact that Silverthorne and Serrano chose the morgue as the setting for their pictures led to many strong reactions by the general public and the critics, who questioned the legitimacy of invading such a delicate space, a location shrouded in the mystery of death with its attendant taboos about handling the dead, a place not even the deceased person's closest relatives and friends would normally have access to.

Another remarkable project dealing with the representation of death is *Body Farm* (2001–2002) by Sally Mann, who photographed the corpses kept by the Forensic Study Facility of the University of Tennessee to study bodily decomposition. Mann, for whom death is a recurring subject, was also harshly criticised for exposing the cadavers, and some critics accused her of being a "grave robber." One writer at the New Yorker described the feeling of the pictures as follows:

> The most morbid pictures contain two kinds of violation. The first, unavoidable if you're set on photographing corpses, is the violation of the privacy and the decency of the dead. In one picture of a decaying corpse, you can't tell a woman's buttocks from her breasts. In another, a man's back has cracked and split apart like dry earth. Another picture shows a shoulder pocked like an orange peel. You want to look away. But Ms. Mann insists on investigating the very surface of the horror.[6]

And on the occasion of an exhibition in London, another critic offered the following reflection.

One does, though, feel like a voyeur when looking at images such as this. They raise the ethical question of whether a person's decision to donate their body to science gives scientists the right, at a later date, to grant Mann permission to photograph that—decomposing—body. (And whether the result should then be displayed as art.)[7]

Mann's intention was to explore the biological process of death itself but at the same time to question the absurdity of negating the human body's inevitable decay, either by denying its occurrence or by preventing it through embalming. Interestingly enough, in a reflection which reveals the difficulties of exhibiting projects dealing with pain and death (even when they come from artists as internationally acclaimed as Mann is), she describes how after four years of work and just four months before it was due to open, the Pace Gallery cancelled her show *What Remains*, which contained pictures from *Body Farm* as well as landscape photographs and portraits. In her reflection, added to the film itself, she suggests that "[the gallery] figured out that it's not going to make Money. I mean, I've known it's not gonna make money since I took the first picture. But that—I mean, that's not—it's still an important show!"[8]

The more recent *Right Before I Die*[9] by photographer Andrew George addresses the issues of pain, illness and death by assembling portraits of dying people along with their descriptions of hopes, dreams and regrets. This project, which clearly revisits the magnificent and celebrated *Life Before Death* by Walter Schels and Beate Lakotta (2003–2004), was completed with the support of the Providence Holy Cross Medical Center in Mission Hills, California, in order to raise awareness about the lives of patients in palliative care and how they face death. Background text described the project and its results as follows:

> Before the exhibition was built, the results of the project were already visible on the Internet. Immediately it generated interest from countries all around the world, more than 150 countries in fact. It inspired hundreds of international reviews. Thousands of comments and letters have been written about 'Right before I die' where people from all over the world have shared thoughts and beliefs as part of a global conversation.[10]

But although the initiative generated interest online, it also provoked controversy of different kinds. While some viewers described the work simply as "beautiful" or "wonderful" (one person's words were "What can one say about such a wonderful tribute to these wonderful people that have taken part?"), others felt the project was inappropriate and took unfair advantage of its subjects ("This photographer is just a talentless, fame-hungry ghoul"; "I wonder if Andrew George will regret milking the dying for profit when he's on his deathbed"; and finally, "Anything to make a few bob—and maybe get famous!!!").[11]

If, as it was argued earlier, the detached art projects tend to provoke more controversy, then the opposite is generally true of the self-referential projects. In other words, the response is of almost absolute acceptance when the artists are directly involved in the story they narrate as a personal experience in pictures (and consequently share through their art work). In this sense, the reactions are similar to the ones received by ordinary users when sharing their images online on either specific memorial sites or social networking sites (SNS) profiles. In most cases, no matter how blunt or explicit the images portraying pain or death are (whether they are contemporary post-mortem photographs, images of the dead in their caskets or portraits of the dying in hospital, among others), the viewers' comments remain compassionate and supportive.[12]

In short, although viewers might argue with an artist's approach to the subject or the nature of the project itself, when that person is portraying and communicating their own reality, this generally takes the edge off most of the controversy, including the issue of whether artists have the right to encroach upon people's privacy or make their private story public. In the same way, photographic art projects dealing with a degenerative illness or death in the family in the artist's inner circle of friends or even the artist's own process of pain or grief represent a whole different approach to these delicate issues and are generally responded to positively, especially when the viewer has experience related to the artist's story.

Furthermore, many of the artists who at some point in their careers delve into issues of pain, illness or death do so as part of a personal grief process. Art projects undertaken in this way to satisfy a personal need to express pain and grief might properly be called "grief projects."[13] Although some works of art may have emerged as a result of the artist's own grief, grief projects deal with pain and grief in a very open, straightforward manner and the process lived by the artist is immediately recognisable. In many grief projects, artists claim to confront their own suffering through the project.

One of the most remarkable projects of this kind in recent years was *Mother's* (2000–2005) by the Japanese artist Miyako Ishiuchi. In this project, which clearly showed the importance of the art process as a means of mediating grief, the artist gathered together portraits of her mother taken earlier in her life and focused on the older woman's skin, revealing its various scars, accumulated over the course of her life, and the ageing of her body. The meaning of these portraits was transformed by their integration in a grief process and the photographs read as maps of the older woman's life on the verge of death, where the photographer seems to find answers to her mother's loss making her skin present. Among these portraits, a group of photographs of Ishiuchi's mother's personal belongings complements the series, including shots in intense colours of her personal lipsticks and other cosmetics. This is combined with phantasmagorical and strangely translucent black and white photographs of her lingerie, which alternately suggest a kind of second skin and ghostly presence, creating the overall effect of an intimate photographic journey that takes in objects which are at the same time highly personal and wholly mundane.

A common part of the experience of bereavement is having to deal with the personal effects of the deceased, in which the grieving person has to decide which objects to preserve as keepsakes and which others to discard as mere junk. About this aspect, Ishiuchi had the following to say:

> I developed the series after Mother died and I was left with her old things. I opened a drawer to find it packed with her underclothes. They looked like fragments of her skin, and I got scared. Although I couldn't use or wear them, or give them away to somebody, I couldn't throw them away like garbage, either. I didn't know what to do. The person who once used them was gone, but she left so many intimate things. It was sad. When I began taking photographs of them, I think I was recording that sense of loss.[14]

Mother's began its life as a reaction of a profound grief resulting from an unexpected death and a complicated relationship between a daughter and her mother, but it took an important step beyond that when Miyako Ishiuchi was elected representative artist for the Venice Biennale in 2005. Because of that, her work found its way to a larger audience and her personal story of grief became an expression of art that needed to be exhibited and that yearned to be shared with the viewer. Ishiuchi also explained how it also changed other things:

> By exhibiting my *Mother's* series in Venice, my mother moved on. She left me behind, and she became art; she stopped being my private mother and became everyone's mother. I saw so many women in the exhibition hall crying at my photographs, and that's when I realized that she wasn't mine anymore. She belonged to everyone.[15]

The example of Ishiuchi's urge to express herself through art in order to understand and overcome a grief process is just one among many. Another factor to consider is that the scope of such art projects often becomes broader either because of the publication of the exhibition catalogue or because the project is published in book form. A good example is an earlier work by photographer Eugene Richards, who dealt with the cancer and death of his wife Dorothea Lynch in the remarkable project *Exploding into Life* (1986). The book brings together fragments of Lynch's diary and her reflections about fighting against cancer, and the photographs by Richards that document the whole process do not only tell of her as a patient but also of him, ultimately, as the bereaved. The work makes a personal story of pain more visible but, just as importantly, it sets out to condemn the patronising treatment of the patients and the dearth of images to help the ill relate to their illness with normality.

> I try to find out what a mastectomy looks like so I call the American Cancer Society. The woman on the other end tells me that books with pictures of cancer treatments aren't considered suitable for non-medical people. And after that, a decision is made: "Maybe you should make photographs of the whole thing," I tell Gene. "If there aren't any pictures of mastectomies, maybe you should take pictures of mine."[16]

In fact, the publication of the work by Edwards provided a groundbreaking example for many individuals living with illness or anticipatory grief and definitely helped to normalise the illness and pain caused by cancer. At the same time the void created by the lack of personal photographs of illness and pain started to be filled, offering visual referents for patients to look at.

Similarly, after she had lost her three-year-old daughter Sophie, artist Belinda Whiting transformed a collection of ordinary family snapshots into a book project to pay homage to her child and normalise the grief process itself, making it visible. In *Sophie's Story* (2011) published with a similar aesthetic to a children's book, the everyday scenes of the little girl are combined with very simple texts that describe the thoughts prompted by the pictures. But some of these texts also describe the most important parts of the story that were not explained in the photographs, such as the moment when the news came that Sophie needed heart surgery, the complications following that and the ultimate death of the protagonist. By narrating these moments in the accompanying text, the ordinary, homey feel of the pictures is re-contextualised and they are transformed into premonitory images of death and grief. As the project description proposes:

> Written to assist the mourning process and confronting loss and grief it is nevertheless a celebratory reflection on a young life. Using simple words and alternating with photographs from the family album, it was written to enhance understanding (particularly for a younger audience) of the reality of a short life that was both ordinary and exceptional.[17]

Sharing Grief Projects Online

Although art books help artists reach a wider audience on a more permanent basis than the strictures of gallery seasons and programming allow, the new millennium has created an unprecedented new scenario. The possibilities offered by the expansion and development of social networks, blogs and the Internet in general have transformed everyday practices for ordinary users[18] and offered the artists new ways of exhibiting their work. By sharing their images online, artists are not only able to reach a potentially unlimited audience but can also receive responses, get constant feedback about their work and communicate with other users directly, in ways beyond anything the art world could ever offer. The increasing presence of new memorial platforms online and the active role of many of the bereaved in websites, blogs and social networks are also changing our relation with death and also the way we mourn[19] (Walter, Hourizi, Moncur, et al. 2012; Walter, 2015), normalising issues of pain, illness and grief and their photographic representations in the online space (Pardo & Morcate, 2016).

Without a doubt, one of the contemporary photographers dealing with pain, illness and grief whose work has acquired greater notoriety as a result of sharing images online is Phillip Toledano. Toledano's work has been clearly marked and transformed by family illness and death, and after the death of his mother he decided to document the time he spent with his father, who suffered from short-term memory loss, until he eventually died. Toledano started *My Ageing Father's Decline: A Son's Photo Journal* as a blog (2006–2010) to get to grips with the fragility of life and the sense that he might be facing the last time shared with his father. As he himself explained in the blog, "It took my mom dying to make me take pictures of my father."[20] And when Toledano started to share these pictures on the blog, the response was massive, showing how completely this kind of project is accepted, met by the gratitude of those who have shared similar experiences and find something in it to relate to.

> After I began to publish these photos, I was surprised and overwhelmed by the way in which people interacted with my story. The site has been viewed by over 1.5 million people, and there are around 20,000 comments. I, personally, have gotten about 10,000 e-mails from people—lovely, honest, extraordinary e-mails. To me, in an odd way, all this is as important as my own story. It was entirely unexpected, and so helpful in dealing with the feelings of loss over my dad.[21]

While some art projects end up as books, in Toledano's case it was the contents of his blog that were finally transformed into a book. After this powerful work, in 2015 Phillip Toledano embarked upon a new grief project (*When I Was Six*), this time tackling a grief process he had repressed (or forgotten) since his childhood when his elder sister Claudia had died in a fire. The idea of working again with such a personal story of pain was inspired by his discovery, on the death of his parents, of a cardboard box containing long-kept hidden belongings of hers. Toledano had never seen this box before, but described it as "an unseen museum to my sister" and which contained "everything related to my sister, her life and her death." The fact that this crucial episode of his life was kept hidden for so many years ("She sort of disappeared from our lives. We never spoke of her again"[22]) was a powerful motivation for Toledano to transform this material into a grief project and narrate in pictures the importance of rediscovering these valuable objects. These included snapshots from the family album, photographs of personal items such a precious lock of hair preserved in a plastic zip lock bag or a carefully folded little dress in a box, which the photographer combined with other pictures to construct space-like landscapes, recreating the only vivid fantasy memories he had for a long period after his sister's death.

To a certain extent, when Toledano manages lost-and-found objects in *When I Was Six*, he does the opposite to what Miyako Ishiuchi did in *Mother's*. She photographed objects in order to obtain the courage to discard them, while his pictures serve to sacralise the objects. At the same time, however, both artists say that the photographs of these objects have been important in their grieving process. Making such a personal story public through his book, exhibitions and interviews forced Toledano to talk about and acknowledge his experience: "This is really the first time I talked about her in about forty years," he said, "and I'm realising what an extraordinary shadow that event cast on my life."[23] In other words, he chose to both literally and metaphorically "open the box" that hid the way the family had faced and managed the grief process and the legacy of their daughter to "get to know her and understand my parents and, I guess, myself."[24]

Another contemporary photographer who has shared his personal story of pain and grief in the form of an art project and on the Internet is Angelo Merendino. Merendino's work exemplifies the effects of sharing an art project online and the new potential those images acquire when uploaded on different online platforms. Furthermore, image sharing has proved to be a powerful tool for the artist in grief in their daily practice of self-expression and interaction with the audience, while it also reflects that person's dual role as a singular artist and ordinary user.

Merendino's Facebook page *My wife's fight with breast cancer* was started in 2011 and is comparable in certain ways to the project by Dorothea Lynch and Eugene Richards. In it, he documents the illness of his wife up to the time of her death from breast cancer. What Merendino makes clear in his project and statement is that he started the project because he needed to make the pain and grief visible. In doing so, he would not only be acknowledged as the bereaved but also use his story as a powerful tool to raise awareness.

> My late wife Jennifer was diagnosed with breast cancer five months after our wedding, and she passed less than four years later. During Jen's treatment we noticed that most people, even those who were closest to us, didn't understand the challenges we faced while living with an incurable disease. At times, sadly, we watched our support group fade in and out of our life. In an effort to communicate with our loved ones, Jennifer allowed me to photograph our day-to-day life. Our hope was that these photographs would show the side of breast cancer that isn't pink ribbons and fundraisers.[25]

Like many artists in grief processes[26] the camera in *My wife's fight with breast cancer* acts as a shield and a mediator through which the artist faces the reality of pain. The need to document has little to do with artistic aspirations; rather, it is the desire to feel useful and busy. For professional photographers, the natural thing to do is photograph:

> Our words were failing as we struggled to make known that we needed help so I turned to the only other form of communication I know - my camera. I began to photograph our day-to-day life. Our hope was that if our family and friends saw what we were facing every day then maybe they would have a better understanding of the challenges in our life. There were no thoughts of making a book or having exhibitions, these photographs were born and made out of necessity.

Here, Merendino expresses a common feeling shared by many grieving artists. The urge to take pictures does not aim at making an artistic profit but is instead indicative of a physical need to capture moments that matter to the artist and find a way to face reality.

> A close friend suggested that I post our story on the Internet and with Jen's permission I shared some of our photographs. The response was incredible. We began to receive emails from all over the world. Some of these emails came from women who had breast cancer. They were inspired by Jennifer's grace and courage. One woman shared that, because of Jen, she confronted her fears and scheduled a mammogram. That's when we knew our story could help others.[27]

Merendino kept posting text and images after his wife's death partly to pay homage to her but also because he understood the power of sharing his work online as an artist and an ordinary person experiencing bereavement who could have an effect on others.

> Jennifer trusted me to make and publish photographs from the most intimate and difficult time in our life. Not long before Jennifer passed I made a promise that the world would know who she was. Technology allows us to make and publish photographs in a fraction of a time that it once took and social networks make sharing our stories easier than ever, offering a chance to reach the world. By sharing our story, our love story, something beautiful has begun to grow out of something so horrible and unfair and if we don't share our experiences with each other, how can we learn to grow and survive?

Another point in common with the work by Lynch-Richards is that the vision of the grieving husband is complemented by the patient's own narrative. In *Exploding into Life*, Lynch's personal narrative blended in with the photographs by Richards, while in Merendino's more contemporary approach to a similar story, Jennifer gave herself a voice by starting a blog called "My life with breast cancer" which she then used to express her fears, the changes she went through and her thoughts, as well as descriptions of how she saw Merendino as a caregiver. One of her posts includes one such portrait of the artist.

> I woke up at 3:30 AM in severe pain! My sweet nurse tried everything she could to take it all away!!!! But nothing… They switched my Meds over to a preservative free version, which seems to be helping a bit…. Sweet Ange is by my side today trying his very best to make me comfortable.[28]

Note, too, that Merendino's blog continues beyond telling his wife's story and, after her death, is progressively transformed into a photographic diary of grief in which the artist keeps posting pictures of his loved one but combines them with other, new pictures that reflect upon his new identity as a widower.

> I've been dreaming about Jen a lot lately. Not sure what it is but I've been feeling like Jen is here with me more often now than ever since she passed. This whole mourning/widower thing is a roller-coaster. (11 July 2013)

By following his SNS profiles and pages, users could retrace the changes in his grief process from one moment to the next and witness the significant impact that grief had on his artistic career. In this sense, it is very interesting to note that the content of most of the viewers' comments was determined by the type of picture Merendino posted. In most of the photographs where we see his wife conducting her everyday battle against cancer or posing next to Merendino in self-portrait mode, the comments are messages of support in which users talk about how powerful the image of love is (among other comments about their experiences of cancer and the value this project has for so many people). On the other hand, the pictures posted on the occasion of an exhibition or a talk led more to comments on the art project itself, but few viewers went into any depth in the discussion of the quality of the photographs or the editing of the work itself. Here, the ambivalence of the artist's role (a photographer *and* an ordinary user) combined with the weight of the issues involved might be enough to make some users refrain from focusing their comments on the artistic side of the project rather than the social value of sharing the images and the story behind them.

Merendino's Facebook page *My wife's fight with breast cancer* is still active. However, over the course of time it has also become a kind of resource page for awareness-raising where visitors can follow his continuing commitment to the memory of his wife, but in which also he lends his voice to other initiatives, patients and caregivers. For example, he has become part of different metastatic breast cancer awareness initiatives.[29] In one of them, he documented the life of the patient Holley Kitchen; and in that capacity he continues to receive users' comments of support, as various messages illustrate (e.g., Jaime Petersen's "I love that you got to be the one to tell Holley's story through pictures. Couldn't admire you both more." Or Wendy Quick's "What a wonderful way you honored your wife in life and in death! You ARE making a difference Angelo!" both posted on 18th October 2015).

Merendino's example is appropriate because of the personal dimension and the way in which his personal narrative and his work blend together and are transformed through his images online. In this sense, it is worth pointing out that the practice of sharing personal images portraying pain, illness and grief is becoming more common among ordinary users but also among artists too. From Instagram to Facebook and Tumblr, and any number of other online platforms, professional artists and photographers are sharing pictures of commissioned work as well as other types of photographs, such as snapshots or more intimate and personal images. One such artist is photographer Terry Richardson, who has used his personal blog to post bluntly direct and powerful pictures of his sick and dying mother in hospital.[30] The announcement of her death, entitled "R.I.P. Annie Lomax, My Mom, 1938–2012," is accompanied a hilariously eccentric portrait of Mrs Lomax from an earlier period. Other shots include a self-portrait of Richardson sitting on his mother's bed and with her ashes in an urn and a shot of the palm of his hand, dusted completely white with those ashes. A series of pictures of bouquets of sympathy flowers sent by different publishers and a photographic journey through the cemetery complete the series.[31] The expressions of support and condolences were numerous: "So sorry for your loss…had seen her on ur tumblr in the past with fab outfits and great attitude. May she RIP…" or "I loved how you captured her. The feeling I got from your images of her along the way is you loved adored and accepted her. When I saw she passed I felt so sad for your loss, arriving at the conclusion your images showed so much love for her."[32]

With comments focusing as often on Richardson's loss as on the photographs themselves, the responses bear witness to how far the boundaries have blurred between the photograph shared as art and the personal picture shared as a means of communicating one's grief to one's peers.

Conclusions

There can be no doubt that online practices and their interaction with digital photography are changing the way we interact with our peers and perceive the world around us. Furthermore, it seems to be changing the way we face pain, grief and death.

The increasing presence online of shared, self-referential images of pain, illness and death is helping to normalise everyday pain and grief. This practice is not solely the prerogative of the artist, given that an increasing number of non-professional photographers and Internet users post personal pictures to share their feelings and interact with their peers. The difference between ordinary users and professional photographers is that, besides being customary users of social media, the professionals also have a powerful ability to use art to make their images express personal stories of pain and grief and to give these images the potential to be solid visual references for others going through similar experiences.

The overwhelmingly positive response that certain art projects have received online is due to the fact that they are self-referential. Most users understand that, no matter how harsh or poignant the pictures might be, they are being used to communicate personal pain and grief, in contrast to other approaches that deal with death and illness from a more detached and detached position.

Through their exhibitions and books, artists can target a varied audience, even while that audience is still limited to those interested in art. They help to normalise delicate issues of everyday pain and to make illness, pain and death more visible. But beyond this, it is through blogs, websites and social media that artists in grief can now not only seek increasingly wider audiences but also develop their projects away from the art world, into something larger and more socially transforming by means of the numerous complex interactions and connections that take place online.

Acknowledgements This chapter stems from the research project *Sharing pain and grief online: the self-referential digital image of illness and death as a means of destigmatization, connection, visibilization and co-presence*, founded by the BBVA Foundation for Scientific Research teams in Digital Humanities (2015–2017).

Notes

1. Batchen, G. *Forget Me Not: Photography and Remembrance* (New York; Amsterdam: Princeton Architectural Press; Van Gogh Museum, 2004); Burns, Stanley B. *Sleeping Beauty: Memorial Photography in America* (Altadena, CA: Twelvetrees Press, 1990); Ruby, J. *Secure the Shadow: Death and Photography in America* (Cambridge, MA: The MIT Press, 1999).
2. Burns, Stanley B. *Sleeping Beauty II Grief, Bereavement and the Family in Memorial Photography American and European Traditions* (New York: Burns Archive Press, 2002); Burns, Stanley B. *Sleeping Beauty III: Memorial Photography: The Children* (New York: The Burns Archive Press, 2011); Linkman, A. *Photography and Death* (London: Reaktion Books, 2011); Morcate, Montse. "Duelo y fotografía post-mortem: Contradicciones de una práctica vigente en el siglo XXI." In *Imagen y muerte*, edited by A. Gondra and G. López (Barcelona: Sans Soleil Ediciones, 2013), 25–45. Online version *Sans soleil* no. 4 (2012): 168–182. http://revista-sanssoleil.com/wp-content/uploads/2012/02/art-Montse-Morcate.pdf (last accessed 05/04/2016).
3. Ariès, P. *Historia de la muerte en Occidente: Desde la Edad Media hasta nuestros días* (Barcelona: Quaderns crema, 2000); Di Nola, A. M. *La muerte derrotada: Antropología de la muerte y el duelo* (Barcelona: Edigrabel, SA para Belacqva, 2007); Mitford, J. *The American Way of Death Revisited* (USA: First Vintage Books Editions, 2000).
4. Sontag, S. *Ante el dolor de los demás*. Torrelaguna (Madrid: Editorial Alfaguara, 2003). Santillana Ediciones Generales, S.L; Reinhardt, M., H. Edwards, E. Dugane, eds. *Beautiful Suffering: Photography and the Traffic in Pain* (Chicago: The University of Chicago Press, 2007).
5. In this sense, grief is understood in wider terms, partly as an acute sense of loss but also as the process experienced by the bereaved. Generally, grief is associated with death but can also be experienced in response to other causes, including degenerative illness, in the form of what is com-

monly termed anticipatory grief (present in many grief projects). See Doka (1989) for an analysis of non-recognised (disenfranchised) grief processes and Cobo Medina (1999) for a detailed classification of grief, including anticipatory, delayed and repressed grief.

6. *The New York Times* photography review by Sarah Boxer (23 July 2004) http://www.nytimes.com/2004/07/23/arts/photography-review-slogging-through-the-valley-of-the-shutter-of-death.html?_r=0 (last accessed on 26/12/2016).
7. Sean O'Hagan, *The Guardian*, June 20, 2010, https://www.theguardian.com/artanddesign/2010/jun/20/sally-mann-family-and-land-review (last accessed 3/1/2017).
8. Sally Mann in the documentary about her life and work *What Remains*, directed by Steven Cantor (2005).
9. Website with information on the project and images at http://www.rightbeforeidie.com/rbid.html (last accessed on 02/01/2017).
10. Press file for exhibition at the Musea Brugge https://www.google.es/url?sa=t&rct=j&q=&esrc=s&source=web&cd=3&cad=rja&uact=8&ved=0ahUKEwjt5MKm6aXRAhWFVRQKHSjcBXwQFggtMAI&url=https%3A%2F%2Fwww.visitbruges.be%2Fpress-file-right-before-i-die-2&usg=AFQjCNHz1HJLRx5TOTJyiWhhIF1K_Go1Qg (last accessed on 03/01/2017).
11. http://www.dailymail.co.uk/news/article-3751568/LA-photographer-s-exhibition-features-portraits-dying-people.html#reader-comments (last accessed on 28/12/2016).
12. Morcate, Montse. "Tipologías y re-mediación de las imágenes de muerte y duelo compartidas en la memorialización online." In *Revista M. Estudos sobre a Morte, os Mortos e o Morrer*, 3, 2017.
13. Morcate, Montse. *Duelo, Muerte y Fotografía: Representaciones fotográficas de la muerte y el duelo desde los usos domésticos al proyecto de creación contemporáneo.* Unpublished PhD thesis (Facultad de Bellas Artes, Departamento de Diseño e Imagen, Universidad de Barcelona, 2014).
14. Itoi, Kay. 2006. "A Daughter's Conversation." *The Japan Times*, Tokio, October 5. http://www.japantimes.co.jp/culture/2006/10/05/culture/a-daughters-conversation/#.Uu5HdbT5Pfs (last accessed on 05/01/2017).
15. O'Brian, J. "On Hiroshima: Photographer Ishiuchi Miyako and John O'Brian in Conversation." *The Asia-Pacific Journal* 10 (2012): 29. See http://japanfocus.org/-John-O_Brian/3709
16. Lynch, Dorothea, and Eugene Richards. *Exploding into Life* (New York: Aperture, 1986), 16–21.

17. Description of the project at the artist's website. http://belindawhiting.co.uk/section/369246_Sophie_39_s_Story.html (last accessed on 29/12/2016).
18. Gómez Cruz, Edgar, and Asko Lehmuskallio, eds. *Digital Photography and Everyday Life: Empirical Studies on Material Visual Practices* (London; New York: Routledge, 2016).
19. Walter, Tony, Rachid Hourizi, Wendy Moncur, and Stacey Pitsillides. "Does the Internet Change How We Die and Mourn? Overview and Analysis." *OMEGA* 64, no. 4 (2012): 275–302; Walter, Tony. "Communication Media and the Dead: From the Stone Age to Facebook." *Mortality: Promoting the Interdisciplinary Study of Death and Dying* 20, no. 3,(2015): 215–232.
20. Rollo Romig for The New Yorker (9 June 2010) http://www.newyorker.com/culture/photo-booth/off-the-shelf-days-with-my-father (last accessed on 30/12/2016).
21. Original text from Phillip Toledano's blog (no longer accessible). Retrieved from Pardo, Rebeca: "Reporting Alzheimer's Through the Lenses of Photojournalism" (International Journalism Week 2014, Sheffield University) (paper).
22. BBC World Service interview with Phillip Toledano, 22 April 2015. https://www.youtube.com/watch?v=jQmhELB2ja4 (last accessed on 21/02/2017).
23. BBC World Serviceinterview with Phillip Toledano, 22 April 2015. https://www.youtube.com/watch?v=jQmhELB2ja4 (last accessed on 21/02/2017).
24. Interview by the *British Journal of Photography* on the occasion of his exhibit in March 2015. http://www.lapietradialogues.org/blog/?p=4018 (last accessed on 15/12/2016).
25. Introduction to the project on the photographer's website. http://www.angelomerendino.com/my-wifes-fight-with-breast-cancer/ (last accessed on 01/01/2017).
26. Morcate, Duelo, Muerte y Fotografia; Morcate, Montse, and Rebeca Pardo. "Grief, Illness and Death in Contemporary Photography." In *Malady and Mortality* (Cambridge Scholars, 2016).
27. *Photo Greater Than 1000: Angelo Merendino at TEDxUSU* published on 18 November 2013. https://www.youtube.com/watch?v=KeT221skphw Part of this talk is transcribed at http://mywifesfightwithbreastcancer.com/our-story/#.WGlH0Gr_qUk (last accessed on 11/01/2017).

28. Posted at https://mylifewithbreastcancer.wordpress.com/2011/11/01/11-1-11/ (last accessed on 03/01/2017).
29. Breast Cancer: A Story Half Told. http://www.storyhalftold.com/about (last accessed on 02/01/2017).
30. 11 September 2012 "My Mom in the ICU," "My Mom's butterfly tattoo."
31. 17 September 2012 "Me holding my Mom's urn on her bed"; "My Mom's ashes on my hand" and 18 September 2012 "Flowers for my Mom from GQ," "Miss You," among others. http://www.terryrichardson.com/diary/#/2012-09/32/0 (last accessed on 02/01/2017).
32. Comments on Terry Richardson's Facebook page on 11 September 2012 (last accessed on 04/01/2017).

Montse Morcate is an artist and Professor of Photography at the University of Barcelona. Her research and art projects deal with photographical representations of death and grief. Recently, she has been a visiting scholar at Columbia University and at the Morbid Anatomy Museum in New York and she has been awarded a research grant on digital humanities by the BBVA Foundation.

7

Pain and the Internet: Transforming the Experience?

Nikki Newhouse, Helen Atherton, and Sue Ziebland

Introduction

In the not so distant past, our conceptualisation of health and illness was relatively simplistic: in illness, we deferred to the expert opinion of a physician, whose higher authority was largely unquestioned. Health information comprised evidence-based facts and figures grounded in hard science, and the subjective, embodied experience of a health problem was hardly acknowledged. A person's awareness of their own health was quite simply secondary to the dominant positivistic medical approach with its onus on quantification and scientific scrutiny.

This model of health and illness fundamentally changed in the early 2000s with the advent of the Internet and the first online search engines. Basic websites featuring lists of information evolved into small but

---

N. Newhouse (✉) • S. Ziebland
University of Oxford, Oxford, UK

H. Atherton
University of Warwick, Coventry, UK

dynamic digital communities of informed consumers. Through this evolution we became proactive *prosumers*, no longer passively receiving our digital diet but actively contributing to it via message boards and discussion forums. The explosion of social media further transformed this digital landscape, offering novel ways to seek out and stay connected to friends, family, and peers. The Internet now shapes many of our daily experiences, including those of health and illness. The emergence of peer-to-peer digital connection has been perhaps one of its most transformative effects, empowering people to use digital resources not only to find health information but also to seek out support and practical advice for self-management, reassurance, encouragement, to compare experiences of treatment and to offer advice and support to others. The traditional doctor–patient dynamic of the not so distant past has been challenged: the patient may now become expert in their own condition through online access to facts and figures and 'alternative' expert information in the form of the experiences of other patients.

This chapter will consider how people who are experiencing chronic physical pain are using the Internet. We examine how immediate access to information transforms the illness experience and how digital resources enable us to express, share, and learn from others' experiences. In particular, we draw on a conceptual review of the potential health effects of accessing other people's experiences online[1] which identified seven domains through which health might be affected, positively and negatively: finding information, feeling supported, maintaining relationships with others, experiencing health services, affecting behaviour, learning to tell the story, and visualising disease. We contextualise these domains and bring them alive by considering them in relation to a collection of qualitative interviews about experiences of chronic pain from an Oxford University archive.

The qualitative interviews include the perspectives of 46 adults with chronic pain from throughout the United Kingdom, who told their stories about living with chronic pain and discussed issues such as searching for a cause, pain management, medication, and impact on lifestyle. A diverse, maximum variation sample was recruited through a variety of sources including support groups, general practitioners, nursing, and allied health professionals and pain specialist consultants. Participants were aged between 24 and 80 years and described being in chronic pain for between 7 months and 45 years. The sample included people who had pain from different origins including injury-related back and neck pain, osteoarthritis, fibromyalgia, post-surgical pain, unexplained abdominal pain and pelvic pain, lupus, multiple sclerosis, post stroke pain, brachial plexus avulsion, and repetitive use wrist and arm pain. Pain related to cancer was excluded. The project was supported by an advisory panel made up of people affected by the health issue, health professionals, academics, and staff from relevant charities. Extracts and further analyses from the interviews have been published elsewhere[2] and on healthtalk. org (www.healthtalk.org/chronicpain). As part of the interview process, participants were asked to talk about how they had used the Internet to find information and support and to communicate with others. People had used the Internet to help them find facts and figures, to find a label for their symptoms, to share ideas about how to manage their pain, and to discuss the merits of different treatment options. Experiential information from others going through something similar helped people to come to terms with a new or changing diagnosis and for learning how to manage pain in daily life.

We draw on the value of first person accounts and the appeal of stories to explore how the Internet may create empowered patients and how the Internet facilitates our collective need to make contact with peers and hear their accounts of pain and illness. We explore the way in which the use of digital resources influences the way people cope with and articulate their pain and the subsequent impact on our engagement with health services.

Finding Information

The first domain that Ziebland and Wyke describe[1] is 'finding information'. Knowledge is power and it is not surprising that many people search for information as soon as they become aware of unusual bodily sensations or symptoms or when they have a searchable label for their embodied experience. A man who had experienced long-term neck and arm pain described how he happened to find a descriptive term that resonated with him while waiting in a doctor's waiting room:

My first introduction to the term, 'chronic pain', came whilst filling time in my GP's waiting room. I saw its Scottish research into chronic pain… I did take that home and had a potter about on the Internet to do a search against chronic pain, and up this site came again.
CP39 (male, aged 38 years)

A woman who had undergone multiple tests and was eventually diagnosed with fibromyalgia talked about the relief of being given a label which could then be used to access information, even if it didn't alter the reality of her prognosis:

So it's actually a release to know, it's got a label, you can't actually do anything about it, it can't be cured but you know there are other people who know what you are talking about which is really helpful.
CP12 (female, aged 47 years)

Online searches for a broad label such as 'fibromyalgia' or 'chronic pain' lead to generic digital resources. Much of the generic information encountered online is presented either in a contextual vacuum or illustrated with one or two patient's stories. It can be hard for people to make sense of such information and apply it to their own circumstances and the significance of what works well, how and for whom can be lost. However, thoughtfully presented digital information is recognised for its ability to integrate, curate, and 'translate' research that may otherwise be inaccessible, as this man points out:

It was an amalgamation of a lot of research that's been done from those accredited books, but it's something that is very readable and quickly understandable, and extremely relevant.
CP39 (male, aged 38 years)

The complexity and uniquely subjective experience of chronic pain means that although generic information can be a good starting point, access to others' experiences is also highly valued for providing face, context, shape, and identity to otherwise abstract facts and figures. Hearing how others have managed their pain can also help people to recognise that action needs to be taken, decide which action to take, and articulate those decisions to health care professionals. A woman who went on to have neck surgery for cervical myelopathy talked about the importance of making informed decisions and being able to explain these choices to health care professionals:

> And I think when you're informed and you go to speak, especially for example if you're trying to determine whether you should go for surgery or not, the more informed you are, the more you can ask of your surgeon and the more, I think perhaps you will feel easier with any decision that you make because it's an informed choice.
> CP15 (female, aged 42 years)

When we make decisions about our health, we draw on a variety of sources of information. Few of us would say that we base all of our decisions upon others' experiences[3] but hearing about how other people have reached important decisions and how they reflect upon the consequences of their choices adds a social and emotional element to an otherwise medicalised process. Experiential information is also valued for its straightforward pragmatism: it's important to know what *works* in real life. Practical tips and advice regarding symptoms and adverse effects of medication, grounded in tried and tested self-management strategies are evaluated alongside information provided by a clinician.

> I use the Internet a lot. I've got a computer at work. I actually found my operation on the Internet. I got more information from the Internet than I did from my GP, from my surgeon.
> CP15 (female, aged 42 years)

Experiential information is powerful because it is vivid; this is also potentially one of its biggest drawbacks. If experiences are presented powerfully yet are not typical or are biased or inaccurate in some way, optimal decisions may be missed or trust broken. Vivid or particularly extreme experiences may not be representative of the unremarkable majority, whose voice may be lost. The Internet is a largely unregulated entity and without conscious and effective efforts at evaluation, all information can be seen as having equivalent status. As such, the work of navigating significant amounts of experiential information may provoke anxiety, especially when accounts offer contradictory advice or information or seem to be driven by commercial or vested interests. Seeking information online could be hard work—people may feel overloaded with information and struggle to make an informed decision.[4]

> Well I find the Internet's really good but I think you do have to be very careful. There's an awful lot of things, I've learnt from other people really on some of these good ones, you know, that some of the websites will say that you can do, if you take this pill it will do this, that and the next thing you know. So I think you have to be really, really careful about what, you know, you listen to and what you don't.
>
> CP34 (female, aged 49 years long-term post-operative pain)

Some people wondered if hearing about other people's experiences was worthwhile, given the uniquely subjective experience of living with pain. For example, a man who had undergone a discectomy following an injury wondered if comparison only served to highlight differences rather than similarities between people:

> The thing that I have noticed about pain is no two people have got the same take on it. I mean my pain isn't the same as somebody else's pain even with a roughly similar injury and I mean pain itself is an intangible.
>
> CP08 (male, aged 53 years)

Feeling Supported

The second domain described by Ziebland and Wyke[1] is 'feeling supported', a widely recognised aspect of online peer communities. Chronic pain and the underlying condition or cause may be a biographically disruptive experience[5] or 'critical situation'[6] challenging one's sense of identity and provoking a fundamental reassessment of one's resources and support networks. Chronic pain is a deceptively simple term yet pain may be unexplained or related to injury, infection, or trauma. The potential complexity and unpredictability of such conditions can be isolating:

I think that chronic pain is quite a, it's quite a lonely sort of thing.
CP34 (female, aged 49)

Going online and participating in peer-to-peer groups or simply reading others' accounts of managing a disrupted life can reduce this isolation and contribute to a sense of being 'normal' or 'differently the same'.[7] The sense of *emotional empowerment*[8] that comes from knowing that we are not alone in our experiences is an important part of feeling more in control, feeling reassured, and simply feeling better. Such empowerment engenders a virtuous circle of receipt and reciprocation in which information and support are actively received and given.[9] Recognition that one is able to offer practical or tangible advice is in itself a recursive and empowering act, indicative of coping and self-efficacy and is acknowledged as being an important part of optimal peer-to-peer functioning.[10] This may be particularly true for those whose condition is rare or who are geographically isolated. Feeling supported is not limited to the sharing of condition-specific information. As this woman points out, although others' advice is critical at times of crisis, there is huge value in being part of an online community where people simply relate to each other as friends who 'happen' to be experiencing shared medical conditions:

> … the other good thing about the Internet is the fact that you meet, and especially for people who are really disabled and can't get out, is that you can have a circle of friends, you know, and talk to people. I mean, if you have a look into some of these forums sort of things, people are just talking about ordinary, everyday sort of things, like things in their back garden, you know, flowers and stuff and I suppose, for some people, that it opens up a new world to them, you know.
> CP34 (female, aged 49 years)

Sharing information is valuable. However, contextualising one's lived experience by engaging with other people's accounts of how they have successfully—or unsuccessfully—managed their chronic pain may provoke anxiety, unrealistic expectations, and feelings of vulnerability, guilt, or inferiority. Finding information that surprises or shocks can be particularly debilitating if encountered while the reader is already feeling vulnerable. The nature of online communication means that certain viewpoints can dominate discussion and, as this woman points out, looking for support online does not necessarily mean that support will be found:

> But sadly I think the more you ask the more you realise that there isn't always an answer and that can be quite difficult because you think, in this day and age of technology, that there will be an answer, there must be an answer, but there isn't always and that's difficult.
> CP15 (female, aged 42 years)

Maintaining Relationships

The third domain concerns relationships, both online and offline.[1] Chronic pain interferes with every aspect of a person's life and the parallel identities of 'patient' and 'person' can be hard to manage; offline relationships can suffer. A woman with abdominal and pelvic pain following an appendectomy explained that her condition affected her old friendships:

> It's like, sometimes I've felt that I've got this secret little world that no one else knows about because you, I don't mention it usually and they don't mention it and it's like we are pretending nothing's actually going on.
> CP16 (female, 25 years)

Friendships can sometimes feel one-sided and people said that pain often dominates their thoughts and puts enormous pressure on the emotional and physical sides of intimate relationships. One woman who had been in a car accident was aware that her persistent pain could be boring or depressing for others to hear about.

> If you are letting off steam with the same person day in and day out, they are going to get tired of it. I think I would get tired of it. So it's trying to strike a balance is also very difficult. Sometimes I have to just shut my mouth when I am in pain.
> CP06 (female, aged 27)

7 Pain and the Internet: Transforming the Experience? 137

Making new friends can be difficult for people in chronic pain who may not want to explain personal limitations. The reality of living with an 'invisible' condition could be stressful and stigmatising. People worried about looking like 'frauds' and, as one man diagnosed with arachnoiditis pointed out, it was easy to feel self-conscious and guilty, even around friends and family:

> And I think even with close personal relationships, when they see you being completely normal because you're in full distraction mode. You are absolutely not thinking about the pain. It's hard for them to believe that there's actually anything the matter with you.
> CP48 (male, aged 61)

Engaging with experiential information from similar others online provides another emotional outlet, helping to separate and maintain what can feel like juxtaposed life roles. People used the Internet to find new ways to successfully manage their 'illness' identity and 'everyday' identity. However, whilst going online to find others is relatively easy, the construction of online relationships differs from offline interactions. Online, people may provide lengthy and intimate detail of their health condition without explanation or justification. This approach may be taken to frame their authenticity as a person living with pain and could also be therapeutic and helpful in forging and integrating a new diagnosis into their life. But it is a strikingly different approach from that found in offline introductions.

Immersion in online, niche support communities can lead, paradoxically, to offline isolation. Opportunities to invest in face-to-face social contact may be lost if people over-invest in online relationships with those who 'really' understand them. A related idea suggests that online activity enables people to refine, personalise, and selectively construct the content and delivery of all the information they receive[11] and, as a result, people are rarely exposed to ideas that challenge their own ways of thinking. This can be damaging within the context of managing dual identities: instead of online and offline relationships supporting each other, they become opposed, with ideas, information and potential misunderstandings entrenched and unchallenged. In addition, if the online help-seeking evokes helpless and gloomy responses, there may be a lack of encouraging 'upward comparisons'[12] A woman with long-term spinal pain said that her condition left her house-bound and reliant on online support. She went online 'for actually some physical contact with other people that have been through the same thing as me' but found that it became important to 'not really give too much of myself to them' explaining

> Because I am quite proactive and positive, I don't want to really dwell on the bad things and I found, in some cases, certainly not in all, but in some cases, the support group seems to be about sharing the bad things rather than sharing strategies and good aspects of management of the pain.
> CP42 (female, aged 24 years)

This was echoed by another woman who had damage to her spinal cord caused by Chiari malformation and syringomyelia. She described the subtle way that negativity pervaded many of her online encounters:

> But I did get the information like the drugs that I am now on from somebody in America from the forum so it was useful as well. But once I was in my higher mood after going onto the Neurontin I decided I didn't need to read two hundred e-mails a day from people who were obviously not very uplifted themselves. So I stopped using the forum.
> CP23 (female, aged 30 years)

Experiencing Health Services

The fourth domain from Ziebland and Wyke's conceptual review concerns how engaging with other people's experiences online can influence how people use health services,[1] for example, whether to have treatment and what treatments to request or avoid.[13] Contemporary neo-liberal health care policies encourage patient choice. Increasingly, people engage with online commentary, feedback, and check other people's ratings of hospitals and clinicians via chat rooms, forums, or social networking platforms. This information can be an effective prompt to actively seek out good treatment and patients are often motivated to maintain a relationship with an individual health care professional. This introduces space for dialogue about information found on the Internet.

An informed patient can approach the health consultation with increased confidence and improve the efficiency, experience, and outcome of the consultation; knowing more about how other people have described their symptoms online can reassure that no action needs to be taken or can offer tips and advice on how to articulate a concern when seeing a doctor. Doctors are becoming used to (and less alarmed by) patients coming in with knowledge gleaned from the Internet. A woman with chronic post-operative abdominal pain said:

> I've found it really helpful to get more information on the Internet and I think doctors are kind of getting more and more used to the fact that their patients will know more about their own condition and a lot of them welcome you coming up with ideas. I mean I've had doctors say to me 'What do you think's wrong with you. Have you managed to find anything on the Internet that you think it could be?' And I think that's good, you know, that they let you have your input.
> CP16 (female, aged 25 years)

Having seen the doctor, people may go online to validate and check advice; this process of engaging with treatment options and alternatives is highly proactive and may help patients to approach difficult situations with more confidence. One woman described how she had satisfactorily managed the process of going in for neck surgery and a subsequent unexpected outcome:

> I mean I knew exactly the procedure I was going in for, I knew why they were doing what they were doing and, when I didn't have the expected result after surgery, I was in fact able to go onto the Internet and find out why that might be the case. And then, when I went to the doctors, went back to the hospital, I was able to ask quite probing questions.
> CP15 (female, aged 42 years)

The Internet often facilitates communication between patient and health care professional. Alternatives to a face-to-face consultation have shown promise in offering continuity of care where numerous face-to-face consultations would be impractical. For patients accessing a pain management unit in a hospital, when given access to a health care professional via email, they reported better communication with the health care professional and better overall satisfaction.[14] The use of telephony by patients with chronic musculoskeletal pain in primary care settings led to both clinical improvement of pain scores and greater satisfaction with pain medication.[15]

People with chronic pain are sometimes prompted to go online in response to unsatisfactory encounters with health care professionals. With no explicit, visible symptoms, people talk about their pain not being taken seriously, or of being aware that their GP sees them as a 'heart sink' patient One woman with osteoarthritis said that her doctor viewed her pain as a uniquely physical symptom, with no acknowledgment of the emotional impact her pain was having on the rest of her life:

> They were only interested in the bit that they were interested in as though I was, you know, I could be chopped up as this is, you know, as though all parts of your body weren't related.
> CP13 (female, aged 63 years)

Lack of interest, time and knowledge are oft-cited reasons for patient dissatisfaction, as one man with long-term back pain explained:

> But I don't seek medical help for pain. I wouldn't, wouldn't even think about it now. It's, it's sort of not in my vocabulary.
> CP30 (male, aged 66 years)

For people with chronic pain, interacting with health care professionals can be a difficult experience.[16] Although many people report a positive response from their doctors to active online information seeking, as many again describe strained clinical relationships and reluctance on the part of health care professionals to acknowledge the validity of information taken from online sources, especially if those sources are peers rather than more traditional medical websites. Engaging with online information may result in overly raised expectations about what can be achieved or it may result in anxiety if particularly vivid or negative stories damage a person's confidence in health care professionals or a particular treatment option. Another concern is that of 'cyberchondria'[17,18]: patients can now research any and all symptoms of a rare disease, illness or condition, and manifest a state of medical anxiety. Over-identification with other people's experiences of illness and treatment can lead to increased use of health services by anxious patients.

Despite evidence to suggest that health care professionals are becoming increasingly used to online searching entering the offline consultation, health care professionals are still learning to understand their patients' interaction with the Internet. They are often sceptical about the quality and content of the information found online.[19] Attempts have been made to classify the way health care professionals respond to the Internet empowered patient. McMullan[20] described three responses to a patient that brings information to the consultation: '(i) the health professional feels threatened by the information the patient brings and responds defensively by asserting their 'expert opinion' (health professional-centred relationship); (ii) The health professional and patient collaborate in obtaining and analysing the information (patient-centred relationship); (iii) The health professional will guide patients to reliable health information websites (Internet prescription)'.

For chronic pain, the reality is somewhere in between, with the interface between health care professional and patient still changing and developing, moving beyond the notion of a patient with a print out. The introduction of newer mediums, such as social media, has impacted on this. For health care professionals the Internet can become a place for them to express their own sentiment about chronic pain conditions, sharing their views via social media. This raises serious questions about how patients might interact with such sites. One example, a site from the US aimed at health care professionals, makes derogatory comments about patients suffering the condition fibromyalgia. This behaviour might be seen to undermine a tool that is useful to patients, in the way that it allows them to find information and feel supported:

End stage fibromyalgia (ESF), affects 1 in 100,000 Americans nationwide. They frequently suffer short employment expectancy, have one of the highest anaphylaxis rates to NSAIDS, and frequently are placed in hospice care, otherwise known as Internet comment forums.
Gomer Blog (2014) (http://gomerblog.com/)

Consequently, the notion of the Internet forum as a safe space for patients might be queried. The increasing role of social media brings into question previously held ideas about the boundaries between health care professional and patient. Both professionals and patients are learning to negotiate these new spaces.[21]

Learning to Tell the Story

The fifth domain from the conceptual review is 'learning to tell the story'.[1] According to Greenhalgh,[22] storytelling may lead to a highly significant improvement in patient enablement in certain chronic disease contexts. The immersive nature of storytelling allows the effective communication of well-timed practical and emotional information. There is a growing realisation that patients and service users are a rich source of health care-related stories that can affect, change, and benefit health care delivery and clinical practice.[23] Learning to tell the story is less about 'what' information is shared and more about 'how' it is delivered, with the onus on learning a new and useful vocabulary. Nutbeam[24] distinguishes between what we now routinely call 'health literacy'—the degree to which individuals have the capacity to obtain, process, and understand basic health information and services needed to make appropriate health decisions—and the consequences of developing a rich and contextualised vocabulary. The ability to tell a pain story *well* serves dual purposes: recursive (re)construction of a coherent narrative may lead to enhanced self-awareness and understanding of our own situation[25] as well as being able to communicate a relevant story concisely to health care professionals. In addition, clear communication may enable us to elicit appropriate support and understanding from friends and family or via online resources. It is relatively easy to share a story on an online forum and doing so can feel empowering, especially if the story provokes positive comment or feedback.

7 Pain and the Internet: Transforming the Experience? 143

People interviewed for the chronic pain project described the difficulty in coming to terms with the reality of pain as a permanent part of their life. The alternative was thought to be pointless anger, aggression, and bitterness that could ruin the person's life and destroy their most important relationships. Constructing a coherent narrative and learning to tell it can be part of the healing process. One woman with lupus described how difficult it was to find the right words to talk about her pain:

> Whereas pain can never really be described, it's either unbearable or its bearable, but to actually describe the pain is a very hard thing to do.
> CP01 (female, aged 56 years)

Another woman with osteoarthritis said that her upbringing and age added to the difficulty of communicating her pain to health care professionals:

> I'm not very good at asking, asking for things I think and also you know when you are in the, I guess I was brought up in an age when doctors were just nearly God and you didn't ask these questions and' I'm a bit better now but I'm still finding, I still find it quite hard when I'm in their presence I suppose.
> CP13 (female, aged 63 years)

People rarely go online with the explicit intention of learning a new vocabulary for their pain; rather, it is part of an accumulative learning process that comes from immersing oneself in relevant information and observations of others' accounts. Bury[26] calls these people's accounts of their experience of illness 'factions', a heavily interpreted combination of fact and fiction subjectively presenting the story in a particular light. Written by people we don't know and will (probably) never meet, encountering multiple stories and multiple ways of telling a story may be confusing. It could even prevent people from forming their own narrative, especially when stories are written in a particularly articulate or compelling manner. There could also be negative consequence if other patients' stories were formulaic or dull. One woman said she was disappointed in the stories she had encountered online: instead of developing a better understanding of her illness and how to communicate it, she found herself inundated by a large amount of well-intentioned but unhelpful email.

> In fairness, I did find out some information because you could just put an e-mail message out and everybody got it so you'd get you know, you could get anything from two replies to two thousand relies replies if everybody had an input in to your particular query. You also got to see other people's queries and replies to them. So you did pick up a lot of information but there was a lot of just sort of patting on the back trying to lift your ego type stuff.
> CP23 (female, aged 30 years)

When people share an illness narrative in a space as public as the Internet, it tends to be with the explicit intention of inviting response. Responses may be negative or non-existent: people may respond with ridicule, correction, or flaming or may simply not respond at all, which can be particularly demoralising.

Visualising Illness

The sixth domain described in the conceptual review concerns the 'visual' presentation of health experiences online.[1] Images on health websites are typically included as part of the overall design or aesthetic framework rather than for any perceived value in the communication of health information. There may seem to be an inherent contradiction in the idea of using imagery in the context of chronic pain, given the 'invisibility' of the condition. People with chronic pain talk about the difficulty of conveying the reality of living with a condition that often has no explicit physical marker. Images of dermatological conditions or weight loss can help people compare and evaluate the outcomes of different treatments or progression of an illness but this is not the case with chronic pain. However, seeing people living with shared conditions can be an important part of feeling supported and reducing perceived isolation; this is particularly pertinent if the experiences that resonate come from people 'like you'. In the context of a condition such as chronic pain, helpful visual images may come in the form of videos of people talking about their condition; practical visual imagery may show how to use walking aids, or the online demonstration of exercise and relaxation techniques which can be useful for modelling helpful activities and behaviours.

The invisible nature of pain leads inevitably to attempts at illustration. Mexican painter Frida Kahlo is considered to be one of the most important 'pain artists', her art often depicting graphically her lifelong struggle with pain following a serious accident in her youth. Contemporary artistic expression such as www.painexhibit.org serves the purpose of facilitating communication between those with chronic pain and a wider audience. The Pain Exhibit (www.painexhibit.org) is an online educational gallery from visual artists who used their personal experiences of pain to create images that are both evocative and troubling. Art elicits an emotional response and this is carried forward in today's digital society, with social media platforms such as Instagram, Tumblr, and YouTube playing an increasingly important role in the visual communication of pain. Expressive imagery such as meme and video allows for the immediate communication of pain in ways beyond that of the factual or biomedical, and often uses blunt sarcasm and humour as a way of conveying sensations that are difficult to vocalise or describe.[27]

Changing Health Behaviours

The seventh and final domain identified by Ziebland and Wyke[1] is the potential effect on health behaviours. The power of the testimonial has long been recognised as a valuable tool in the art of persuasion. The advertising industry uses personal stories to generate sales; a technique adopted in the field of health behaviour change. Health websites offering advice and support on a variety of public health concerns such as weight loss, smoking cessation, or practising safe sex routinely provide narratives as a way of motivating behaviour change by breaking down resistance and the tendency to distance or discount oneself from unwelcome messages.

Interview participants often said that although their lives were now limited, they had found ways of making their daily tasks more manageable. Some had learned from others how to manage their activities and minimise pain by prioritising tasks, setting goals, and pacing. People had also picked up tips to make tasks easier. However, living well with chronic pain is not simple. Hearing about how others have managed a problem or a concern can build confidence and self-efficacy, which can in turn prompt healthy shifts in behaviour. In some cases, hearing about other people's experiences may reinforce unhelpful or unhealthy behaviours. Some websites contain messages that contradict or challenge medical advice while others feature stories of behaviour change that are so extreme as to be demoralising. Reading about people who have 'overcome' a condition in order to run a marathon, for example, can inadvertently reinforce the idea that small steps towards healthier behaviours are not worth trying.

Instead, people described learning to integrate their pain into a new lifestyle that may involve learning as much about which behaviours cannot be changed as which behaviours can. Interview participants talked about learning to accept that pain was going to be a part of their lives and that certain activities were no longer going to be possible. A man who experienced chronic pain following a spinal stroke talked about how persisting with the idea that he could perform certain activities was demoralising and he felt that he had wasted a lot of time trying to return to the person he was before his stroke:

> And that was a major problem at the beginning with me. It took me two years, at least two years, to come to terms with that. Because I was always making a target of getting back to the way I was. It's totally unrealistic. It's never going to happen.
> CP32 (male, aged 57)

Reading online about how others had come to accept their diagnosis helped people to develop a new set of behaviours. One woman talked about how important it was for her to accept that the reality of her back pain meant that she would not return to her old job:

And most of all it was the hardest part, but I accepted that I had this damn back, and that I would have it for the rest of my life but there was a life with back pain and once I'd accepted that I'd, I just got on with my life and I've got a different life now.
   CP17 (female, aged 63)

Discussion

In this chapter we have drawn on a conceptual review, featuring seven domains through which access to other patients' experiences online might influence health. The seven domains from the review have been considered in relation to a secondary analysis of narrative interviews conducted with people living with chronic pain. We have found that the domains encapsulate the online motivations and experiences of people with chronic pain. The domain concerned with 'visualising' the condition might be considered less relevant in chronic pain but (as other contributions to this volume demonstrate) the experience of pain can be represented through art, sound, and literature. Resources drawing on these media could help fulfil the potential of this domain in chronic pain by communicating the effects of the experience of chronic pain to others.

To contextualise these observations further, contemporary health care narratives suggest that the role of patient comes with certain responsibilities as well as rights.[28] Those living with one or more long-term, chronic conditions may find that 'patient-centred care' is increasingly synonymous with 'self-motivated patient empowerment'. The Chronic Care Model emphasises the centrality of the informed and activated patient who engages readily with a 'prepared and proactive practice team',[29] consistently self-managing conditions through a set of 'lifestyle' choices, such as diet and exercise. The wider biomedical model underlines this, with its inherent expectation that compliance with the advice given by the physician regarding self-care 'ought to be adhered to as a matter of individual responsibility and duty'.[30]

Online resources increasingly play a central role in this conceptualisation of the patient as a responsible and proactive *consumer*[31] of health care information. Indeed, with the advent of Web 2.0 and 3.0 communication media, the patient as consumer has evolved into patient as *prosumer* of e-health resources, accessing, exchanging, and producing health information through multifaceted participation in online self-management, self-expression, and 'peer-to-peer healthcare' practices.[32]

Access to digital resources is a uniquely powerful tool in the context of living with chronic illness in general: Grant et al.[33] found that 44% of 900 patients with type 2 diabetes used the Internet to retrieve health information; half of cancer patients have used the Internet at least once to access information about their condition,[34] with patients under the age of 50 years more likely to do so. Unsurprisingly, living with an invisible or contested illness is a particularly important motivator to engage with online resources.[35] However, those living with one or more chronic diseases are generally less likely to have access to online information[32] and older, male online adults of low socioeconomic status are less likely to engage in e-health activities in general.[36] Nonetheless, those who are online are significantly more likely to be highly engaged with others via social media, blogs, and online health discussion groups.[32] It is not merely the presence of a particular chronic illness that determines the frequency and type of Internet use, but rather the total number of chronic conditions that a person lives with.[37]

People who do have Internet access and skills can now engage in a complex bricolage of clinical and digital information gathering, using online resources for their 'privacy, immediacy [and] …variety of perspectives'.[38] In the context of chronic pain, this bricolage acts as a bridge between the worlds of clinical and personal expression. People with chronic pain may use social media platforms such as Facebook, YouTube, and Tumblr to address the 'epistemic injustice' of clinical communication[27] and create safe spaces online. Social media plays a unique role in pain communication, providing immediate, relevant, and private opportunities for people to transform 'flesh into words'.[39] The ongoing disruption of chronic illness[5] is addressed by the creative remobilisation of new resources, and social media platforms allow for what Goffman (1978)[40] termed the 'polyvocal' expression of pain, often through expression of humour and sarcasm via flexible, visual, and written media. Social media in particular allows people with chronic pain to connect with others on their own terms and feel 'differently the same'.[7]

People with chronic pain actively work towards gaining knowledge to create a new sense of normal and make better-informed decisions, often going online to seek out information to help them confirm that they can trust and rely upon their physician.[41] Surveys suggest more than one-third of chronic pain patients seek out health information related to their condition online and that 60% of patients feel more confident in the information provided online than provided by their physician.[42]

This is problematic, not least because of the evidence base, which suggests that the majority of information accessed online by patients is of poor quality.[43] Patients' digital practices are a general concern for many health care practitioners: there is a risk of harm if patients rely on digital resources to self-diagnose or ignore a health professional's recommended treatment in favour of 'cures' found online. A number of studies have concluded that around 40% of UK patients or carers who attend an outpatient clinics have used the Internet to search for health-related information (ibid) and that those managing chronic illness are more likely to access health care-related Internet sites than others.[32] Thirty nine per cent of patients with chronic pain have searched the Internet for pain-related information.[43] It therefore makes sense that chronic pain patients form an important subset of those who are likely to be looking at and for online information and that digital resources relating to chronic pain need to be fit for purpose.

Patients with chronic pain are highly motivated to seek out online information, but digital pain-relevant information is often considered difficult for patients, particularly adolescent patients, to read and can often be judgemental of particular coping strategies.[44] Rather than leaving patients to navigate the Internet alone in the hope of finding the 'right' information, it is increasingly recognised that health care professionals should routinely ask patients (of all ages and social backgrounds) if they, or a family member on their behalf, use the Internet. For those with access, the health professional should recommend reliable sites as a starting point. Surveys demonstrate that up to three-quarters of patients attending a Pain Centre would like to receive information about relevant websites from medical staff.[45]

Peer-to-peer platforms are an important tool for communicating the experience of pain, enabling the Internet to be used as 'a communications tool, not simply an information vending machine'.[32] The Internet has changed many people's experience of health and illness and will likely continue to do so as new platforms and applications are developed in coming years. Chronic pain can have a dramatic limiting impact on people's lives—relationships with health professionals, family, colleagues, and friends can all be jeopardised by a suite of conditions that prevent activities yet are frustratingly invisible to others.[2] People with chronic pain face multiple challenges, including the need to come to terms with the fact that a cure, or even, in many cases, an explanation, is unlikely. When people in pain hear this news from health care professionals, they often feel that they are not being taken seriously, or that they are not being believed or are suspected of malingering. Hearing the same message from other people with pain, who have found ways to manage similar conditions, can be a more acceptable conduit as well as providing the benefits of information, practical tips, social support, and human connection. Exposure to another person's lived experience of pain offers an opportunity for simple yet powerful comparison: it can help boost confidence or allay fear and also allows a person to engage fully with their own diagnosis by comparing and evaluating symptoms, treatments, and outcomes with others. Hearing about how others have managed a similar situation may impact on how a person views their own condition and offer a new and viable way of approaching it. For these reasons, we believe that the use of the Internet to support peer-to-peer community connections is unlikely to diminish.

Acknowledgements We are grateful to Dr Clare Dow (nee Mortimer) who conducted the original study for HealthTalk.org on experiences of chronic pain. Her research was supported by Queen Margaret University College Edinburgh and The Health Foundation.

Notes

1. Ziebland, Sue, and Sally Wyke. "Health and Illness in a Connected World: How Might Sharing Experiences on the Internet Affect People's Health?" *The Milbank Quarterly* 90, no. 2 (2012): 219–249.

2. Dow, Clare M., Patricia A. Roche, and Sue Ziebland. "Talk of Frustration in the Narratives of People with Chronic Pain". *Chronic illness* 8, no. 3 (2012): 176–191.
3. Entwistle, Vikki Ann, Emma F. France, Sally Wyke, Ruth Jepson, Kate Hunt, Sue Ziebland, and Andrew Thompson. "How Information About Other People's Personal Experiences Can Help with Healthcare Decision-Making: A Qualitative Study". *Patient Education and Counseling* 85, no. 3 (2011): e291–e298.
4. Hart, Angie, Flis Henwood, and Sally Wyatt. "The Role of the Internet in Patient–Practitioner Relationships: Findings from a Qualitative Research Study". *Journal of Medical Internet Research* 6, no. 3 (2004): e36.
5. Bury, Michael. "Chronic Illness as Biographical Disruption". *Sociology of Health & Illness* 4, no. 2 (1982): 167–182.
6. Giddens, Anthony. "Agency, Structure". In *Central Problems in Social Theory* (Macmillan Education UK, 1979), 49–95.
7. Mazanderani, Fadhila, Louise Locock, and John Powell. "Being Differently the Same: The Mediation of Identity Tensions in the Sharing of Illness Experiences". *Social Science & Medicine* 74, no. 4 (2012): 546–553.
8. van Uden-Kraan, Cornelia F., Constance H. C. Drossaert, Erik Taal, Bret R. Shaw, Erwin R. Seydel, and Mart A. F. J. van de Laar. "Empowering Processes and Outcomes of Participation in Online Support Groups for Patients with Breast Cancer, Arthritis, or Fibromyalgia". *Qualitative Health Research* 18, no. 3 (2008): 405–417.
9. Lin, Tung-Ching, Jack Shih-Chieh Hsu, Hsiang-Lan Cheng, and Chao-Min Chiu. "Exploring the Relationship Between Receiving and Offering Online Social Support: A Dual Social Support Model". *Information & Management* 52, no. 3 (2015): 371–383.
10. Dennis, Cindy-Lee. "Peer Support Within a Health Care Context: A Concept Analysis". *International Journal of Nursing Studies* 40, no. 3 (2003): 321–332.
11. Negroponte, N. "Being Digital. New York, Alfred A. Kopf" (1995).
12. Salzer, Mark S., Steven C. Palmer, Katy Kaplan, Eugene Brusilovskiy, Thomas Ten Have, Maggie Hampshire, James Metz, and James C. Coyne. "A Randomized, Controlled Study of Internet Peer-to-Peer Interactions Among Women Newly Diagnosed with Breast Cancer". *Psycho-Oncology* 19, no. 4 (2010): 441–446.

13. Bruce, Bonnie, Kate Lorig, Diana Laurent, and Philip Ritter. "The Impact of a Moderated E-mail Discussion Group on Use of Complementary and Alternative Therapies in Subjects with Recurrent Back Pain". *Patient Education and Counseling* 58, no. 3 (2005): 305–311.
14. Ruiz, Irene Solera, Guadalupe Poblaciòn García, and Irene Riquelme. "E-mail Communication in Pain Practice: The Importance of Being Earnest". *Saudi Journal of Anaesthesia* 8, no. 3 (2014): 364.
15. Kroenke, Kurt, Erin E. Krebs, Jingwei Wu, Zhangsheng Yu, Neale R. Chumbler, and Matthew J. Bair. "Telecare Collaborative Management of Chronic Pain in Primary Care: A Randomized Clinical Trial". *JAMA* 312, no. 3 (2014): 240–248.
16. Briones-Vozmediano, Erica, Carmen Vives-Cases, Elena Ronda-Pérez, and Diana Gil-González. "Patients' and Professionals' Views on Managing Fibromyalgia". *Pain Research and Management* 18, no. 1 (2013): 19–24.
17. White, Ryen W., and Eric Horvitz. "Cyberchondria: Studies of the Escalation of Medical Concerns in Web Search". *ACM Transactions on Information Systems (TOIS)* 27, no. 4 (2009): 23.
18. Starcevic, Vladan, and Elias Aboujaoude. "Cyberchondria, Cyberbullying, Cybersuicide, Cybersex: 'New' Psychopathologies for the 21st Century?" *World Psychiatry* 14, no. 1 (2015): 97–100.
19. Anderson, James G., Michelle R. Rainey, and Gunther Eysenbach. "The Impact of CyberHealthcare on the Physician–Patient Relationship". *Journal of Medical Systems* 27, no. 1 (2003): 67–84.
20. McMullan, Miriam. "Patients Using the Internet to Obtain Health Information: How This Affects the Patient–Health Professional Relationship". *Patient Education and Counseling* 63, no. 1 (2006): 24–28.
21. Atherton, Helen, and Azeem Majeed. "Social Networking and Health". *The Lancet* 377, no. 9783 (2011): 2083.
22. Greenhalgh, Trisha. "Chronic Illness: Beyond the Expert Patient". *BMJ: British Medical Journal* 338, no. 7695 (2009): 629–631.
23. Haigh, Carol, and Pip Hardy. "Tell Me a Story—A Conceptual Exploration of Storytelling in Healthcare Education". *Nurse Education Today* 31, no. 4 (2011): 408–411.
24. Nutbeam, Don. "Health Literacy as a Public Health Goal: A Challenge for Contemporary Health Education and Communication Strategies into the 21st Century." *Health Promotion International* 15, no. 3 (2000): 259–267.

25. Carlick, A., and Francis C. Biley. "Thoughts on the Therapeutic Use of Narrative in the Promotion of Coping in Cancer Care". *European Journal of Cancer Care* 13, no. 4 (2004): 308–317.
26. Bury, Mike. "Illness Narratives: Fact or Fiction?" *Sociology of Health & Illness* 23, no. 3 (2001): 263–285.
27. Gonzalez-Polledo, Elena. "Chronic Media Worlds: Social Media and the Problem of Pain Communication on Tumblr". *Social Media + Society* 2, no. 1 (2016): 2056305116628887.
28. Powell, John, Nikki Newhouse, Anne-Marie Boylan, and Veronika Williams. "Digital Health Citizens and the Future of the NHS". *Digital Health* 2 (2016): 2055207616672033.
29. Wagner, Edward H., Susan M. Bennett, Brian T. Austin, Sarah M. Greene, Judith K. Schaefer, and Michael Vonkorff. "Finding Common Ground: Patient-Centeredness and Evidence-Based Chronic Illness Care". *Journal of Alternative & Complementary Medicine* 11, no. supplement 1 (2005): s-7.
30. Rogers, Anne, and Nicola Mead. "More Than Technology and Access: Primary Care Patients' Views on the Use and Non-use of Health Information in the Internet Age". *Health & Social Care in the Community* 12, no. 2 (2004): 102–110.
31. D'Auria, Jennifer P. "Googling for Health Information". *Journal of Pediatric Health Care* 26, no. 4 (2012): e21–e23.
32. Fox, Susannah, and Kristen Purcell. *Chronic Disease and the Internet* (Washington, DC: Pew Internet & American Life Project, 2010).
33. Grant, Richard W., Enrico Cagliero, Henry C. Chueh, and James B. Meigs. "Internet Use Among Primary Care Patients with Type 2 Diabetes". *Journal of General Internal Medicine* 20, no. 5 (2005): 470–473.
34. Basch, Ethan M., Howard T. Thaler, Weiji Shi, Sofia Yakren, and Deborah Schrag. "Use of Information Resources by Patients with Cancer and Their Companions". *Cancer* 100, no. 11 (2004): 2476–2483.
35. Berger, Magdalena, Todd H. Wagner, and Laurence C. Baker. "Internet Use and Stigmatized Illness". *Social Science & Medicine* 61, no. 8 (2005): 1821–1827.
36. Kontos, Emily, Kelly D. Blake, Wen-Ying Sylvia Chou, and Abby Prestin. "Predictors of eHealth Usage: Insights on the Digital Divide from the Health Information National Trends Survey 2012". *Journal of Medical Internet Research* 16, no. 7 (2014): e172.

37. Ayers, Stephanie L., and Jennie Jacobs Kronenfeld. "Chronic Illness and Health-Seeking Information on the Internet". *Health* 11, no. 3 (2007): 327–347.
38. Cotten, Shelia R. "Implications of Internet Technology for Medical Sociology in the New Millennium". *Sociological Spectrum* 21, no. 3 (2001): 319–340.
39. Gere, Cathy, and Bronwyn Parry. "The Flesh Made Word: Banking the Body in the Age of Information". *Biosocieties* 1, no. 1 (2006): 41–54.
40. Goffman, Erving. "Response Cries". *Language* (1978): 787–815.
41. Nettleton, Sarah, Roger Burrows, and Lisa O'Malley. "The Mundane Realities of the Everyday Lay Use of the Internet for Health, and Their Consequences for Media Convergence". *Sociology of Health & Illness* 27, no. 7 (2005): 972–992.
42. Bailey, S. Jeffrey, Diane L. LaChapelle, Sandra M. LeFort, Allan Gordon, and Thomas Hadjistavropoulos. "Evaluation of Chronic Pain-Related Information Available to Consumers on the Internet". *Pain Medicine* 14, no. 6 (2013): 855–864.
43. Corcoran, Tomás B., Fran Haigh, Amanda Seabrook, and Stephan A. Schug. "The Quality of Internet-Sourced Information for Patients with Chronic Pain is Poor". *The Clinical Journal of Pain* 25, no. 7 (2009): 617–623.
44. Henderson, Ellen M., Edmund Keogh, Benjamin A. Rosser, and Christopher Eccleston. "Searching the Internet for Help with Pain: Adolescent Search, Coping, and Medication Behaviour". *British Journal of Health Psychology* 18, no. 1 (2013): 218–232.
45. de Boer, Maaike J., Gerbrig J. Versteegen, and Marten van Wijhe. "Patients' Use of the Internet for Pain-Related Medical Information". *Patient Education and Counseling* 68, no. 1 (2007): 86–97.

Nikki Newhouse is a researcher with the Health Experiences Research Group in the Nuffield Department of Primary Care Health Sciences, University of Oxford. She has a particular interest in human–computer interaction and interdisciplinary design for well-being.

Helen Atherton is Assistant Professor of Primary Care Research at the University of Warwick. She specialises in digital health care with a focus on how communications technologies and the Internet impact on patients and health care professionals.

7 Pain and the Internet: Transforming the Experience?

Sue Ziebland is Professor of Medical Sociology in the Nuffield Department of Primary Care Health Sciences, University of Oxford, Director of the Health Experiences Research Group, and an National Institute for Health Research (NIHR) Senior Investigator. Sue is a medical sociologist with increasing focus on qualitative research. She has a particular interest in how people use the Internet in relation to their health.

8

Photography and Mental Illness: Feeding or Combating the Stigma of Invisible Pain Online and Offline

Rebeca Pardo

Introduction

This chapter analyses the role of images in the creation of stigmatized iconographies of illness, particularly of mental health, and how photographs can be mediators in the process of de-stigmatization and a medium of communication and connection between peers, one without language limits. It is the result of an investigation that has already originated several publications in the fields of art and communication. The chapter will focus on ethical questions about how images can feed or combat stigma, which can be analysed using the style guides for journalists proposed by patient and relative associations. These guides expose some linguistic appreciations about how to write in a more sensible and conscious way to avoid incorrect and dangerous denominations that contribute to stigmatization and prejudice and their proposals will be "translated" to the visual field in this chapter. The aim is to interrogate the role of the photographer in the social perception of illness and pain, to consider whether

---

R. Pardo (✉)
University of Barcelona, Barcelona, Spain

the "scientific" representation of diseases in which pain is invisible is as "objective" as it claims to be, and to determine whether the people behind the diseases and symptoms have been ethically represented.

This chapter provides a conceptual and historical context based on an interdisciplinary theoretical framework through discussion of themes including illness narratives, stigma, anticipatory grief and show how contemporary media narratives imply that the patient is responsible for the malady. Some illnesses, particularly mental ones, are especially sensitive to these implications, as the pain is understood to exist only in the patient's mind. This chapter also focuses on explaining some essential concepts in order to understand the difference between autobiography and self-reference and its implications in the generation and sharing of images, and in defining the role of the *affiliative look* in the emotional connection of strangers through a photograph. By tracking the evolution of the relationship between photography and illness, this text addresses longstanding questions about the role of the photographer and the objectivity of the scientific representation of illness. Medical photographs and photojournalism have played a central role in creating a visual representation of illness since the nineteenth century, offering an external vision, and for some themes such as AIDS or mental health, they focused attention on the most radical, violent and extreme symptoms and patients. Nevertheless, not every illness image has stigmatizing effects, and this chapter will examine why some seem to dehumanize the patient while others do not have the same effect. For this reason, the research is focused on framing how mental health images can affect the public image and the social perception of those patients. It will be necessary to explain how these kinds of diseases have been represented by doctors and photojournalists to better understand what patients and relatives have been doing online in recent years.

If doctors' representations focus primarily on illness and its symptoms, photojournalists have started using images to denounce the poor conditions in some mental health institutions. Photographs of a few exceptional cases have contributed to the stigmatization of a bigger, invisible group by depicting them as dangerous, violent, linked to crime, fear, danger and pain. There was an important step towards de-stigmatization of the illness in 1961, when three books[1] stated that mental health patients were human beings with an illness. Since that time, "madness" can be seen as a cultural product.

The other important step was the anti-psychiatry movement that also had its influence on photojournalism (or vice versa), and in the last years, it is important to consider the images of photojournalists with relatives affected with mental health problems, as they have been contributing to humanizing the iconography on this theme. Nevertheless, taking into account that pain is invisible in mental illness and frequently chronic, the supposed objectivity of its possible visual representation is questionable.

Due to the difficulty that patients and caregivers have in gaining a hearing or space for their point of view in the "traditional" mass media, this study focuses on how they have begun to represent themselves online with digital photography, particularly phonography,[2] on a daily basis as normal people with an illness, instead of just containers of a dangerous or worrying disease. When these images are shared on social networks and the Internet (via Instagram, blogs, etc.), they reach a level of public visibility that was unthinkable before. In this context, new photographic practices are emerging that are linked with experiences of co-presence and the generation of new kinds of communities for sharing experiences and communicating between peers.

Previous Research

My previous research about visual narratives of illness online and offline,[3] demonstrated that self-referential and autobiographical images are usually explicit about pain and medical issues. They may also be related to some anticipatory grief elements, particularly in Alzheimer's cases, that go beyond what is usually considered "photographable".[4] Consequently, such images are sometimes classified as morbid or narcissistic.

In contrast with this idea, we demonstrated[5] that these kinds of images, including photographs, videos and films, fight against stigmatization and solitude by showing the more human side of illness. They depict the vulnerable intimacy of patients and their families/friends in homes and hospitals at good and bad times, with scars and marks of pain on their bodies, but sometimes also with smiling faces. Tenderness, happiness, fun and good cheer are almost combative elements in the struggle against an illness and the fight for life and in the normalization and humanization of how some chronic, terminal or degenerative illnesses are viewed.

Thus far, my previous studies have analysed the most "normalizing" snapshots of illness shared on social networks (such as Instagram) by patients, associations and carers. In this context, they have also focused on the explicit self-referential images of illnesses and diseases integrated into family, domestic or intimate narratives offline and online and compared them with other visual narratives produced by an external photographer.

Efforts to represent the person (not the illness) and his or her context and needs in a trustworthy, honest way occurred more frequently towards the end of the twentieth century. Such images avoid the most radical, stigmatizing representations and redress the absence of images of "normal" everyday moments that a patient also has over the course of a chronic, degenerative or terminal illness.

The quantity and presence of such images is increasing significantly, mostly in self-referential or autobiographical projects, by *photographers*[6] who work with illness narratives within their own lives or those of their families. These pioneering images, along with the new digital and online context, have contributed to changing poses and clichés of "happy families" by including in domestic narratives scenes of pain and sorrow, as well as boring or inconsequential daily moments that together are essential for understanding the many dimensions of their lives beyond their symptoms and illnesses.

Ethical Questions

To understand the role of images in the creation of stigmatized iconography of illness in general, and of mental health issues in particular, this section provides a discussion of the ethics of the visual representation of the human being behind the pain, pathologies and symptoms.

The first issue is to clarify whether the images of violence, marginalization and danger offered by the media represents the real group affected by mental illness. According to the World Health Organization,[7] one in four families has at least one member affected by a mental disorder, and these people are more likely to be victims of human rights violations, stigma and discrimination.[8] However, the *Confederación Española de Agrupaciones de Familiares y Personas con Enfermedad Mental* (FEAFES), referring to WHO data, points out that less than 3% of the population diagnosed with schizophrenia or with other psychoses commit acts of violence.[10] Mental health problems therefore affect a high and increasing percentage of the world's population, but only a very low percentage of those with mental health problems will commit acts of violence. However, since journalism usually requires an item to be "newsworthy" for it to be published, the photographs of these exceptional cases are often the only ones in the media, and cause people to disproportionately associate the disease with crime and violence. As the Style Guide to Mental Health and Media proposed by FEAFES[11] emphasized, the representation in the media of people with a mental illness is usually negative and linked to the role of "disturbed" individuals. They are identified as feared, rejected, causing shame and punished, and the illnesses and pain they generate are associated with embarrassment. FEAFES also points out that when the information is positive it is covered from a paternalistic perspective that highlights needs and ignores capabilities.

Mental health representation (visual or not) is a complex, sensitive field in which any generalization, simplification or use of symbols or terminology can be dangerous. In this respect, Emily Martin, a recognized anthropologist who has suffered the stigmas of having this type of disease, defends the term "mental illness" against "madness" in her book *Bipolar Expeditions: Mania and Depression in American Culture*.[12] Similarly, the Alzheimer's Foundation in Spain[13] states that the term "dementia" has a very negative connotation and should only be used in medical vocabulary. FEAFES[14] supports the use of diagnosis or "having" a specific disorder versus terms that label people with the adjective of their condition such as "schizophrenic", "anorexic" or "manic".

All these linguistic factors can be translated into the visual field: a more realistic and everyday image of the "patient" as a person who "has" mental health problems should be provided, instead of the stereotyped, frozen image of a "mad" person. This is more or less what people with personal involvement with these illnesses are doing on social networks, blogs and reportages, but there is more work to be done on the awareness of media and professionals who approach the problem from the outside.

The aforementioned FEAFES Guide[15] highlights the widespread use of negative images in the mass media that do little to normalize mental illness. It mentions illustrations in which people with these disorders are represented as passive beings with no social interactions that transmit feelings of pity, loneliness, isolation or imbalance.[16] As Susan Sontag pointed out, there is a grammar and even an ethics of vision.[17]

FEAFES[18] recognizes that photographing mental illness is complex because it involves pathologies that do not change the physical aspect of the person. Therefore, mental illnesses are called 'invisible' diseases. Furthermore, Depardon[19] explains that when *manicomios* were closed and he asked what would happen next, the answer was "there are no more photos to be taken, the prison is chemical now". Elaine Scarry's reflections about the unsharability and resistance to the language of pain[20] can be added here. The lack of scars or marks may have helped the most sensationalist or metaphorical images to occupy the visual void in the visual representation of mental illness.

As Kirkman[21] mentions, media coverage of Alzheimer's disease and other dementias is framed within three major discourses: biomedicine, ageing and gender, which all contribute to the stereotyping of the malady. The current active presence of people with mental illnesses online could fill an important gap highlighted by FEAFES: the underrepresentation of patients as a source of information.[22] Therefore, FEAFES asks the media to avoid illustrating information with the most "extravagant" or disturbing images, those that focus only on social isolation and lack of productivity, or those that directly arouse compassion or rejection.[23]

In this attempt to change the public image of mental health, there are some interesting initiatives, such as the AGIFES (Guipuzcoan Association of Relatives and People with Mental Illness) photo contest entitled *Enfoca la Salud Mental*,[24] which held its fifth edition in 2016 and rewards new ways of observing mental health and looking at people with mental and family problems.[25]

Theoretical Frameworks

As mentioned in the introduction to this chapter, two main concepts can be used to refer to these images/projects: self-reference and autobiography. It is important to explain the difference between them. "Self-referentiality" (referring to oneself) has been used for general purposes since the beginning of this study, because it is a broader concept that can easily encompass all the works examined. According to the paradigm proposed by Philippe Lejeune,[26] the main character, narrator and author must be the same person for a project to qualify as autobiographical. Depending on the illness, most of the photographs and projects analysed were created and shared by relatives and caregivers, who are usually the authors and even the narrators of the photo-stories. Nevertheless, the main character is usually someone else: the patient. Carers and relatives are secondary characters or extras in these visual narratives, which are therefore not always autobiographical but self-referential, if only because the authors' refer to their own family, fear, love, loss, pain or even anticipatory grief in Alzheimer's cases, for example.

There are some exceptions, in which the patient is the author, narrator, main character and the person responsible for the social media profile. It could be said that different visual narratives are generated by different illnesses. Some online profiles of people with eating disorders or epilepsy try to normalize living with these illnesses. In contrast, autobiographical artwork by David Nebreda, a Spanish artist with schizophrenia, is really painful and questioning.

These photographic practices are emerging within the theoretical frameworks of other disciplines such as anthropology, sociology, psychiatry or psychology, in which illness narratives[27] or important concepts such as "anticipatory grief"[28] have been developed. For the purposes of the analysis below, the definition of stigma proposed by Goffman is particularly relevant: "situation of the individual who is disqualified from full social acceptance".[29] This is complemented by Foucault's idea[30] that every system of social control produces some waste that could be described as unclassifiable and irreducible.

The degenerative process of the patient, the chronic invisible pain or the irremediableness of the disease can prove to be stigmatizing elements that compound the health problem by adding social isolation. Certain contemporary narratives exacerbate the problem by implying that the patient is responsible for the malady.

According to Elizabeth Peel,[31] the mass media contribute to the creation of opinions in this area by publishing portraits of people with an illness that are designed to enhance the image of "innocent victims" or people that "deserve their fatality" (or destiny). Kirkman[32] agrees, concluding that people living with Alzheimer's disease are represented as victims of both illness and health services. Peel considers that British newspapers are augmenting the concept of individual responsibility for the development of illnesses such as dementia by suggesting that these diseases could be prevented by a change in behaviour or lifestyle. Responsibility for the disease is thus attributed to the individual rather than public health. This is just one example of how new elements are added to social intolerance that increase its area of influence every time that the margins of what can be considered deviant behaviour are extended.[33] This is what enables certain kinds of patients marginalized as "mad" or "AIDS sufferers" to become, at certain points in time, the great scapegoats of a society and culture that needs to feel "clean" and "disciplined".[34] Javier Moscoso also refers to this idea of blaming patients with mental illness and holding them responsible when he explains that in traditional clinical medicine pain can be observed in its physical manifestations, but in mental illness the patients cannot understand the circumstances that seem to make them responsible for their own suffering. This is because their experience refers to something that seems to exist only within the limits of their consciousness.

In this context, those who need to express their pain, suffering or fears can find a medium of communication in the image via social networks and blogs, where they can contact peers who understand their feelings, suffering and pain without judging them.[35] In these kinds of connections, what Marianne Hirsch called the "affiliative look" plays an important role. This is a process by which a person is involved with the image of a stranger due to the ability to adapt it to his/her own family narrative by recognizing his/her own experiences in the photograph.[36] Visual narratives of illness do not have language barriers, so immediate connections can be made whose characteristics are similar to those of Maffesoli's[37] emotional communities, Benedict Anderson's[38] imagined communities and even Van House's[39] communities of practice.

As Gail Weiss[40] suggests, in this type of affiliative look, the image becomes a place of mediation, negotiation and commitment. This is particularly important when autobiographical or self-referential images of an illness are shared in which the important thing may not be the information or the specific people that are depicted, but the complicity and negotiation with their own processes of pain with strangers or acquaintances who are far away. In this way, illness images shared online can become scenarios or spaces of relationship.

In order to understand the role of these visual exchanges, another complementary concept is "co-presence", as proposed by Ito.[41] People exchange messages that Ito has called "ambient virtual co-presence"[42] such as "I'm tired", "I'm sick", "I'm going to bed" or "it hurts" through messaging apps on smartphones. For Ito, the aim of these types of experiences is not explicit communication, since she clarifies that between friends and relatives who are frequently in contact, the messages do not need to be interesting or informative to be worth sending.

Photography and Illness

The themes that society considers "photographable" have changed over the brief history of photography. The visual representation of illness is a case in point. Montse Morcate[43] explains that in other periods, such as the Victorian era, very sick or dead people were often photographed for the family to keep a memory of them. However, these images were soon dropped from family albums and even from the media, apart from on exceptional occasions.

The complex relationship between photography and pain, illness and death was widely analysed by Susan Sontag[44] who suggests that to photograph is to participate in the mortality and vulnerability of another person.[45] It is important to understand that "ours" will be photographed in a more dignified, caring way,[46] and this is why the point of view in photography changes when illness is photographed by relatives and patients instead of by external professionals (doctors or photojournalists).

The other interesting question is why some illnesses are stigmatized and others are not. For Sontag, the real problem of illness is not only the possibility of a death sentence, but the consideration of the "obscene".[47] In some cases, Sontag coincides with the aforementioned theories of Peel[48] and Kirkman[49] on patient blame. For her, heart disease does not have the same connotations as tuberculosis because it relates to a mechanical failure that is not taboo or embarrassing, while tuberculosis suggests the presence of resonant, terrible life processes.[50] This is why the most frightening illnesses are those that seem not only lethal, but also dehumanizing.[51] This is particularly important in the mental health cases that will be analysed, and in other cases, such as AIDS or breast cancer, that will not be discussed in detail here.

Mental Health Images

The maladies that generate this type of new visual narratives are often chronic, terminal or degenerative. The main issues addressed in this paper up to this point have been common to all diseases in general, but mental illnesses, and especially Alzheimer's, have been chosen for a more in-depth case study. This section describes some specific characteristics that differ from other visual narratives, such as those generated by AIDS that are more centred on activism, or those of breast cancer that are focused on the demand for women's agency over their bodies.

The Beginning: Medical Images

The nineteenth century was an era marked by the works of pioneers in physiognomy, morphopsychology and anthropometry. In positivist criminology, the traits of criminals were considered extremely relevant, and photography became an important element for forensic, judicial and/or social protection activities. This approach is important to contextualize medical (psychiatric) photography, as it was the beginning of attempts to catalogue the physical characteristics that were most closely related to the human mind. This opened the door for psychiatrists to try to classify or characterize mental illness in a comprehensive visual way.[52] The situation reached the point that Yayo Aznar Almazán[53] even compared it with representations of botanical species, and Julie L. Mellby[54] described it as a form of "orthography of the physiognomy in motion".

After the invention of photography in the nineteenth century, some hospitals and/or doctors acquired basic photographic equipment so that they could produce images to illustrate their research or medical texts. The first photographs of this kind were calotypes made by psychiatrist Hugh Welch Diamond[55] in 1851 in England. Rafael Huertas points out that after Diamond's work, the practice of photographing patients became widespread and medical records and files began to incorporate photographs as another piece of information.[56]

Subsequently, photography was widely used in psychiatry studies. La Salpêtrière already had a well-equipped photography studio in 1878,[57] and at this time the Bellevue Hospital in New York also had a photography department. The result of these first experiences was the publication of a treatise on medical photography in 1893 entitled *La photographie médicale: application aux sciences médical et physiologiques* by Albert Londe.[58] However, Michele Ristich de Groote[59] comments that "the exacerbated symptoms of Charcot's great hysteria disappeared when doctors stopped believing in them: there are ways of being insane in each culture".[60]

Rafael Huertas considers that the *Revue photographique des Hôpitaux* published in Paris in 1869 was a pioneering work in the use of photography for clinical purposes. He identifies the relevance of this type of images in medicine for scientific communication and teaching as an important technical novelty that revolutionized medical iconography. Photography offered a supposedly objective image that reinforced the ideal of clinical observation by being able to capture it through a message without a code.[61] For this reason, photographs were considered to have predictive and probative capacity (both diagnostic and pedagogical) in an era in which the anatomo-clinical method was applied, not always successfully, in cases of mental disorders. The objectivity or scientific value of these images will not be analysed here, but Yayo Aznar[62] believes that Diamond himself may have manipulated his images to enhance the visible features of the disorder so that they better fit the definitions of the illness.

These images made by doctors and institutions, which could be retouched and manipulated, along with paintings by artists with mental disorders that were frequently selected or valued by their doctors, were the basis of the model of classic visual representations of mental health problems.

In his book about the cultural history of pain, Javier Moscoso[63] refers to the counter-intuitiveness and even absurd nature of the unconscious pain of mental illness. He emphasizes how after the most extraordinary or visible manifestations of hysteria, for example, there was chronic, constant and intractable pain that was not visible or "observable" in traditional clinical medicine. It could be added that it was also invisible to photography.

Photojournalism: Critical Images

Photojournalism, documentaries, scientific or academic publications or even cinema fiction have been nurtured by this iconography, which leads us to another important question: how the stigmatized image of mental health has been constructed. Since the beginning of photojournalism, photography has been used as a medium to denounce certain situations, such as the bad conditions in some mental health institutions.

In this section, we will mention some cases of this kind of photography as *social criticism*. Examples include the images of treatments applied to patients with mental health problems at Pilgrim State Hospital, Brentwood, NY, which Alfred Eisenstaedt published in LIFE in 1938, or images showing the bad conditions of mental hospitals in the US, published by Albert Q. Maiseldel in 1946 in the Reader's Digest.[64]

In his cultural history of psychiatry, Rafael Huertas[65] identified 1961 as the year that changed the theoretical framework of mental illness. In this year, three essential books were published by Foucault,[66] Goffman,[67] and Szasz[68] stating mental health patients were not "crazy", but were human beings with an illness who had families, rights and feelings. These books paved the way to seeing "madness" as a cultural product and to the emergence of "anti-psychiatry". Questions and denials of the scientific nature of psychiatric institutions that were observed in subsequent photographic reports are an undeniable consequence of these theories and the surrounding social debate. At that time, asylums began to be seen and portrayed as spaces for surveillance, discipline and social control.

As a result of this new vision of mental illness, the award-winning photographer Raymond Depardon carried out probably one of the best-known projects on this subject when he photographed Italian psychiatric institutions between 1977 and 1981. The images were recently published in the book *Manicomio*.[69] Depardon's black and white photographs are hard and painful. They represent daily life inside these psychiatric institutions until they were closed by a law passed in Italy in 1988. These photographs contributed to the general image of mental health associated with the ideas that Sontag mentioned: obscene, embarrassing and dehumanizing processes of illness and pain. Nevertheless, the images were instrumental in changing the institutions and the conditions for patients. Depardon[70] states in his book that Franco Basaglia told him "the psychiatric hospital made them [the patients] that way", but that it was too late for them and that exactly the same situation could be found in France and America. Basaglia asked Depardon to take the photographs because "otherwise people won't believe us". Oscar Martínez and Luisa Serrulla[71] even question whether the aforementioned Italian law would have existed without the support of social documentary photography or *concerned* photography.

The problem is not the intention of these photographs or the fact that they were published, but that for many years these dramatic images (along with the medical ones) were practically the only available public representation of mental health and this had consequences. Socially critical images related to health issues continue to be published today, although in recent years they are often produced in the institutions of cultures farther from the Western world. For example, the award-winning José Manuel Cendón Docampo photographed psychiatric hospitals in the DRC, Burundi and Rwanda in 2006. In these cases, the image of mental illness is linked to centres of internment, reclusion and/or detention and to cases of serious illness in which inmates are photographed writhing in pain or absent, violent, and/or outside of society, images that can also be seen in cinema.[72]

In order to normalize and humanize the public image of mental health institutions, using a less dramatic approach, some contemporary photographic projects have been undertaken inside residences. The focus is not pain or the problems of institutions, but patients as people with a life and emotional needs inside the hospital or residence. These images help to open the debate about current care policies by focusing on the effects they can have on somebody's life. This is the case of *Into Oblivion: Documenting Memory Loss from Alzheimer's*,[73] by Maja Daniels, who took colour photographs recording the experience in an Alzheimer's ward over a three-year period. The images humanize the inmates with suggestive photographs, such as those of patients standing in front of the ward's locked exit door. Another example is *The faces of Alzheimer's*, by Cathy Greenblat, which focuses on the activities of Alzheimer's patients.

Other contemporary reportages have chosen to personalize the experience by following a specific person, as in *Living with Alzheimer's*[74] by Kenneth O'Halloran. In these photographs, we see Angel Serrano and his family in less isolated, less conventional images of mental illness, including wide-angle shots and close-ups outside and inside the house. However, there are some elements taken from the traditional vision of mental health, such as aberrant angulations and contrasted black and white. Illness in this case is not the focus; the emphasis is on family care and solidarity.

As Allison M. Kirkman[75] points out, the mass media could reduce the stigma associated with dementia, but a recent study suggests that newspapers maintain "conventional characteristics" of this illness, as these examples confirm.

However, the vision of mental illness in photojournalism or documentary, especially in cases of Alzheimer's disease, is closer and less obscure when the photographers are the patient's friends or relatives. In recent years, there have been numerous examples of projects carried out by photographers or filmmakers who show in their images their personal experiences as caregivers of a family member with mental health problems.

A clear example of this kind of images is the award-winning reportage *Never let you go*[76] by Alejandro Kirchuk. In his colour images, Kirchuk shows his grandfather caring for his grandmother who has Alzheimer's disease, focusing attention on the carer and the affection with which he looks after his wife at home. A similar situation is depicted in *The Sandwich Generation*, made by Julie Winokur and Ed Kashi (filmmaker and photographer) in 2006 when they brought Winokur's father to live at their home because of dementia problems. Daily life with the two children of the couple and the completely dependent 83-year-old is shown in a photo reportage and a documentary video that focuses again on the family context, caring and moments of normal life, such as going to the supermarket or eating. Other contributions to the de-stigmatization and normalization of the public image of mental illness are being made by publications showing the experience of well-known people who have diseases such as Alzheimer's. A clear example is the book *Pasqual Maragall Mira*,[77] comprising images from a mobile phone taken every day by Pasqual Maragall, a Catalan politician,[78] since he has been suffering from Alzheimer's disease.

Blogs, Social Networks and Common Users

Due to the difficulty patients and caregivers have in accessing as authorized voices or references the "traditional" mass media to offer themselves a different image of these illnesses, it is important to value how patients, caregivers, relatives, friends and the organizations and associations of which they are members have begun to use digital photography, particularly phonography and the Internet (blogs and social networks) to represent themselves publicly on a daily basis. The aim is to disseminate a less dramatic and closer/human public visual representation of their lives.[79] As a consequence, they can now show themselves as normal people with an illness (not just a dangerous or worrying illness "containers" or "carriers") in domestic, familiar images that connect with others through the aforementioned "affiliative look".[80]

Self-referential and autobiographical images showing daily life with illnesses such as epilepsy or dementia can easily be found on social networks like Instagram, usually with tags such as #awareness. The tagged images increase the visibility of the diseases and make it easy to connect with other common Internet users who may share similar experiences of pain or illness through the photographs and comments. As they are anonymous and I would like to preserve identities for ethical reasons, I will not provide any names here, but we can give an example of a blog that was so successful that it was also published as a book.[81] The blog was called *My Aging Father's Decline: A Son's Photo Journal* by photojournalist Phillip Toledano, who is a clear example of a carer of a parent with Alzheimer's disease (in his case from 2006 until 2010). The harshness of this malady, which often involves anticipatory grieving, and the dedication it demands from caregivers (usually relatives) seems to create the context for sharing daily experiences with the disease, grief and pain in blogs. Phillip Toledano is a photographer, so his photographs are particularly interesting: highly contrasted and in colour, they show us tender moments or funny pictures of an increasingly physically exhausted father. The blog generated an enormous response; Phillip Toledano himself stated that he was surprised and overwhelmed by the way people interacted with his story. The site was viewed by over 1.5 million people and there were around 20,000 comments, as well as about 10,000 personal emails.[82]

There are other examples, such as the blogs that were cited in previous publications[83]: *Diario de un cuidador* (Diary of a caregiver)[84] by Pablo A. Barredo, *Mi vida con el Alzheimer* (My life with Alzheimer's)[85] by Isabel Cordero, or *Ella, el Alzheimer y yo* (She, Alzheimer's and me)[86] by Carmen Lucena. All of the authors were caregivers of relatives with Alzheimer's disease.

Stereotypes are broken in these images taken and shared by relatives or patients online. Even daily situations such as medicalization or hospitalization can be tackled with humour. Selfies, family and domestic images and close-up shots of pills or drippers show people's everyday experiences with illness and pain without drama, fleeing from passivity, isolation and stereotypes. The patients and their families are shown as normal people who love and are loved, who cry and laugh, who suffer, have fun and go to the doctor, which normalizes the public image of mental illness and its context. In line with Sontag's aforementioned concerns, perhaps these pictures contribute to dignifying pain and humanizing people affected by mental health problems.

Conclusions

The relationship between photography and illness goes back many years, to the early days of the medium. At this time, institutions and medical professionals used photography, which was considered more objective than words, to catalogue, study and reinforce their theories and carry out research. However, there is clear evidence that the images were manipulated to make the illustrations fit the theories. These medical images provided the basis for the visual representation of certain diseases, such as mental illnesses, which were completed with the contributions of mass media (and cinema).

Thus, in medical journals and in mass media, the patient has been classified as a carrier of illnesses and has not been photographed as a person but as a sick body. In addition, due to the characteristics of the visual medium and the invisibility of pain in mental health, the images usually reflect patients' suffering from the most visually accessible, dramatic and "spectacular" symptoms of their maladies. This, along with some film clichés, creates an iconography of certain patients as violent, dangerous, unstable or passive people, which in turn contributes to their stigmatization.

Patients as human beings going about their daily lives were poorly represented until the arrival of the Internet and social networks. Digital photography and the Internet have democratized and expanded the public image of disease, putting the visual narration of their circumstances into the hands of the patients themselves and their closest circle, which dignifies their experience. Hence, an interesting change is underway in the emitters, actors, media and messages involved in the visual communication of illness and the expression of pain.

This vision of illness is closer to the daily reality of thousands of people, is more humanized, and better portrays the lives of those affected. However, this vision is still not projected in many media. Some organizations and associations have designed their own contests and guides that could help to foster change in this area.

News related to persons with diseases should be represented with appropriate images that are not morbid or extravagant, do not focus only on the negative, incurable or compassionate side, and do not mix mental health, or any other disease with another type of disability or with crime and violence.

Finally, the growing number of "domestic" images shared online by people who lead quite normal lives with bipolar disorders, schizophrenia or epilepsy contribute to humanizing and normalizing the previous image of the "mad". The authors of these images are trying to fight against the vision of obscene pain and stigma by showing patients as simple human beings with a medical problem. They suffer and laugh, have jobs and families and share with us the right to dignity and control of their own (good) image.

Acknowledgements This chapter was supported by the research project: "*Sharing pain and grief online: the self-referential digital image of illness and death as a means of destigmatization, connection, visibilization and co-presence*", funded by the Ayudas Fundación BBVA for Scientific Research teams in Digital Humanities (2015–2017).

Notes

1. Foucault, Michel. *Historia de la locura en la época clásica II* (México, DF: Fondo de cultura económica, 2010); Foucault, Michel. *Historia de la locura en la época clásica I* (México DF: Fondo de cultura económica, 2011); Goffman, Erving. *Internados. Ensayos sobre la situación social de los enfermos mentales* (Buenos Aires: Amorrortu, 2001); Szasz, Thomas S. *El mito de la enfermedad mental* (Buenos Aires: Amorrortu Editores, 1994).
2. Term used for mobile phone photography.
3. Morcate, Montse, and Rebeca Pardo. "Grief, Illness and Death in Contemporary Photography". In *Malady and Mortality: Illness, Disease and Death in Literary and Visual Culture*, edited by Helen Thomas, 245–254 (Cambridge Scholars, 2016); Pardo, Rebeca. "La Autorreferencialidad en el arte (1970-2011): El papel de la fotografía, el vídeo y el cine domésticos como huella mnemónica en la construcción identitaria". PhD Thesis, Universitat de Barcelona, 2012; Pardo, Rebeca. "Documentales autorreferenciales con Alzheimer (O cómo la enfermedad del olvido impulsa la recuperación audiovisual de la memoria y la

historia)". In *Actas Congreso Internacional Hispanic Cinemas: En Transición. Cambios históricos, políticos y culturales en el cine y la televisión* (Madrid: UC3M, 2013); Pardo, Rebeca. "Self-Reference, Visual Arts and Mental Health: Synergies and Contemporary Encounters". In *Auto/Biography Yearbook 2013* (Bulwell Lane, Basford, Nottingham: Russell Press, 2014), 1–21; Pardo, Rebeca. "Imágenes de la (des)memoria: narrativas visuales autorreferenciales del Alzheimer en Barcelona". Master Thesis, Universitat de Barcelona, 2014. Accessed January 15, 2017. http://hdl.handle.net/2445/66651; Pardo, Rebeca. "Reporting Alzheimer Through the Lenses of Photojournalism". Conference in *International Journalism Week 2014*, University of Sheffield, Sheffield, UK, November 13–14, 2014; Pardo, Rebeca. "Imágenes autorreferenciales de la enfermedad online: visibilidad y copresencia". *Actas de II Conferencia Internacional de Comunicación en Salud*, 2015. Accessed January 15, 2017. http://e-archivo.uc3m.es/handle/10016/22271; Pardo, Rebeca. "Enfermedad mental, fotoperiodismo e Internet: hacia una visión más humana y normalizadora". *adComunica. Revista Científica de Estrategias, Tendencias e Innovación en Comunicación* 13 (2017): 83–109. doi:10.6035/2174-0992.2017.13.6; Pardo, Rebeca, and Montse Morcate. "Illness, Death and Grief: The Daily Experience of Viewing and Sharing Digital Images". In *Digital Photography and Everyday Life*, edited by Edgar Gómez Cruz and Asko Lehmuskallio (Routledge, 2016), 70–85.
4. Pardo, Rebeca. "La muerte como final de proyecto: La representación de la muerte en narraciones autorreferenciales fotográficas "online" y "offline" de enfermedad". *Revista M. Estudos sobre a Morte, os Mortos e o Morrer*, 2, vol. 1 (2016): 379–400. Accessed February, 19, 2017. http://www.revistam-unirio.com.br/la-representacion-de-la-muerte-en-narraciones-autorreferenciales-fotograficas-de-enfermedad-contemporaneas/
5. see note 3.
6. "Photographers" in this text includes professionals and common users of mobile cameras (smartphonography): if any distinction is required, it will be specified.
7. WHO. *Invertir en Salud Mental* (Switzerland: Organización Mundial de la Salud, 2004), Accessed January, 15, 2017. http://www.who.int/mental_health/advocacy/en/spanish_final.pdf
8. WHO, *Invertir en Salud Mental*, 4.
9. Spanish Confederation of Groups of Relatives and People with Mental Illness.

10. FEAFES. *Salud mental y medios de comunicación. Guía de estilo. Segunda Edición Actualizada* (Madrid: Confederación Española de Agrupaciones de Familiares y Personas con Enfermedad Mental [FEAFES], 2008), 11. Accessed January 15, 2017. https://consaludmental.org/publicaciones/GUIADEESTILOSEGUNDAEDICION.pdf
11. FEAFES, *Salud mental y medios de comunicación. Guía de estilo. Segunda Edición Actualizada* (Madrid: Confederación Española de Agrupaciones de Familiares y Personas con Enfermedad Mental (FEAFES), 2008), 13. Accessed January 15, 2017. https://consaludmental.org/publicaciones/GUIADEESTILOSEGUNDAEDICION.pdf
12. Martin, Emily. *Bipolar Expeditions: Mania and Depression in American Culture* (Princeton; Oxford: Princeton University Press, 2009).
13. Fundación Alzheimer España http://www.alzfae.org/ (last visited 04/01/2017).
14. FEAFES. *Salud mental y medios de comunicación. Guía de estilo. Segunda Edición Actualizada* (Madrid: Confederación Española de Agrupaciones de Familiares y Personas con Enfermedad Mental [FEAFES], 2008), 23. Accessed January 15, 2017. https://consaludmental.org/publicaciones/GUIADEESTILOSEGUNDAEDICION.pdf
15. FEAFES. *Salud mental y medios de comunicación. Guía de estilo. Segunda Edición Actualizada* (Madrid: Confederación Española de Agrupaciones de Familiares y Personas con Enfermedad Mental [FEAFES], 2008). Accessed January 15, 2017. https://consaludmental.org/publicaciones/GUIADEESTILOSEGUNDAEDICION.pdf
16. FEAFES. *Salud mental y medios de comunicación. Guía de estilo. Segunda Edición Actualizada* (Madrid: Confederación Española de Agrupaciones de Familiares y Personas con Enfermedad Mental [FEAFES], 2008), 14. Accessed January 15, 2017. https://consaludmental.org/publicaciones/GUIADEESTILOSEGUNDAEDICION.pdf
17. Sontag, Susan. *Sobre la fotografía* (Madrid: Santillana Ediciones Generales, 2006), 15.
18. FEAFES. *Salud mental y medios de comunicación. Guía de estilo. Segunda Edición Actualizada* (Madrid: Confederación Española de Agrupaciones de Familiares y Personas con Enfermedad Mental [FEAFES], 2008), 14. Accessed January 15, 2017. https://consaludmental.org/publicaciones/GUIADEESTILOSEGUNDAEDICION.pdf
19. Depardon, Raymond. *Manicomio* (Paris: Fondation Cartier pour l'art contemporain, 2013), 11 from last w.n.

20. Scarry, Elaine. *The Body in Pain. The Making and Unmaking of the World* (New York: Oxford University Press, 1985), 4.
21. Kirkman, Allison M. "Dementia in the News: The Media Coverage of Alzheimer's Disease". *Australasian Journal on Ageing* 25 (2006): 74–79.
22. FEAFES. *Salud mental y medios de comunicación. Guía de estilo. Segunda Edición Actualizada* (Madrid: Confederación Española de Agrupaciones de Familiares y Personas con Enfermedad Mental [FEAFES], 2008), 15. Accessed January 15, 2017. https://consaludmental.org/publicaciones/GUIADEESTILOSEGUNDAEDICION.pdf
23. FEAFES. *Salud mental y medios de comunicación. Guía de estilo. Segunda Edición Actualizada* (Madrid: Confederación Española de Agrupaciones de Familiares y Personas con Enfermedad Mental [FEAFES], 2008), 21. Accessed January 15, 2017. https://consaludmental.org/publicaciones/GUIADEESTILOSEGUNDAEDICION.pdf
24. Focus on Mental Health.
25. AGIFES, *V Concurso de Fotografía Enfoca la salud mental*, 2016, 1. Accessed January 15, 2017. http://www.agifes.org/sites/default/files/concursos/AGIFES_Bases_concurso-fotografia_Enfoca-la-Salud-Mental2016.pdf
26. Lejeune, Philippe. *Le pacte Autobiographique* (Paris: Seuil, 1975); Lejeune, Philippe. "El pacto autobiográfico, veinticinco años después". In *Autobiografía en España: un balance*. Proceedings of an International Congress of the Philosophy Faculty of Córdoba, 25–27, October, 2001 (Madrid: Visor Libros, 2004), 159–172.
27. Kleinman, Arthur. *The Illness Narratives: Suffering, Healing, and the Human Condition* (New York: Basic Books, 1988); Couser, G. Thomas. *Recovering Bodies. Illness, Disability and Life Writing* (Madison, WI: The University of Wisconsin, 1997); Frank, Arthur W. *The Wounded Storyteller. Body, Illness, and Ethics* (Chicago: The University of Chicago Press, 1995).
28. Gatto, Marceio E. *Duelo Anticipado y Conspiración del Silencio*. Conference, *I Jornada Argentina de Psicooncología*, 2004. Accessed October 23, 2016. https://docs.google.com/viewer?a=v&pid=sites&srcid=ZGVmYXVsdGRvbWFpbnxncnVwb2RlZXN0dWRpb2Fcm9wb3N8Z3g6MzFiMzE1MjUwOTYyOTliZQ; Kübler-Ross, Elisabeth and David. *Kessler, Sobre el dol i el dolor* (Barcelona: Edicions 62, labutxaca, 2010).
29. Goffman, Erving. *Estigma. La identidad deteriorada* (Buenos Aires: Amorrortu, 2006), 7.

30. Michel. *El poder psiquiátrico: Curso en el Collège de France (1973-1974)* (Buenos Aires: Fondo de Cultura Económica, 2007).
31. Peel, Elizabeth. "'The Living Death of Alzheimer's' Versus 'Take a Walk to Keep Dementia at Bay': Representations of Dementia in Print Media and Carer Discourse". *Sociology of Health & Illness* 36, no. 6 (2014): 885–901. Accessed January 15, 2017. http://doi.org/10.1111/1467-9566.12122
32. Kirkman, Allison M. "Dementia in the News: The Media Coverage of Alzheimer's Disease". *Australasian Journal on Ageing* 25 (2006): 74–79.
33. Huertas, Rafael. *Historia cultural de la psiquiatría: (Re)pensar la locura* (Madrid: Los Libros de la Catarata, 2012), 42.
34. Huertas, Rafael. *Historia cultural de la psiquiatría: (Re)pensar la locura* (Madrid: Los Libros de la Catarata, 2012), 44.
35. Pardo, Rebeca. "Imágenes autorreferenciales de la enfermedad online: visibilidad y copresencia". *Actas de II Conferencia Internacional de Comunicación en Salud*, 2015. Accessed January 15, 2017. http://e-archivo.uc3m.es/handle/10016/22271; Pardo, Rebeca, and Montse Morcate. "Illness, Death and Grief: The Daily Experience of Viewing and Sharing Digital Images". In *Digital Photography and Everyday Life*, edited by Edgar Gómez Cruz and Asko Lehmuskallio, 70–85 (Routledge, 2016).
36. Hirsch, Marianne. *FAMILY FRAMES. Photography, Narrative and Postmemory* (USA: Harvard University Press, 2002), 93.
37. Maffesoli, Michel. *El tiempo de las tribus* (Barcelona: Icaria, 1990).
38. Anderson, Benedict. *Comunidades Imaginadas: Reflexiones sobre el origen y la difusión del nacionalismo* (México: Fondo de Cultura Económica, 2011).
39. Van House, Nancy A. "Feminist HCI Meets Facebook: Performativity and Social Networking Sites". *Interacting with Computers* 23, no. 5 (2011): 422–429. Accessed January 15, 2017. http://www.academia.edu/7507760/Feminist_HCI_meets_Facebook_Performativity_and_social_networking_sites
40. Weiss, Gail. "Drawing the Affiliative Look". *Drawing Out 2010: Proceedings of the International Transdisciplinary Conference on Drawing*, RMIT, Melbourne, VIC, (2010): 1–8. Accessed January 15, 2017. http://hdl.handle.net/10536/DRO/DU:30068742
41. Ito, Mizuko. "Intimate Visual Co-Presence". *The Pervasive Image Capture and Sharing Workshop*, Ubicomp (2005). Accessed January 15, 2017. http://www.itofisher.com/mito/archives/ito.ubicomp05.pdf

42. Ito, Mizuko. "Intimate Visual Co-Presence". *The Pervasive Image Capture and Sharing Workshop*, Ubicomp (2005): 1. Accessed January 15, 2017. http://www.itofisher.com/mito/archives/ito.ubicomp05.pdf
43. Morcate, Montse. "Duelo, Muerte y Fotografía. Representaciones fotográficas de la muerte y el duelo desde los usos domésticos al proyecto de creación contemporáneo". Master Thesis, Universitat de Barcelona, 2014, p. 158.
44. Sontag, Susan. *La enfermedad y sus metáforas y El sida y sus metáforas* (Buenos Aires: Taurus, 2003); Sontag, Susan. *Sobre la fotografía* (Madrid: Santillana Ediciones Generales, 2006); Sontag, Susan. *Ante el dolor de los demás* (Madrid: Santillana ediciones generales, Alfaguara, 2007).
45. Sontag, Susan. *Sobre la fotografía* (Madrid: Santillana Ediciones Generales, 2006), 32.
46. Sontag, Susan. *Ante el dolor de los demás* (Madrid: Santillana ediciones generales, Alfaguara, 2007).
47. Sontag, Susan. *La enfermedad y sus metáforas y El sida y sus metáforas* (Buenos Aires: Taurus, 2003), 123.
48. Peel, Elizabeth. "'The Living Death of Alzheimer's' Versus 'Take a Walk to Keep Dementia at Bay': Representations of Dementia in Print Media and Carer Discourse". *Sociology of Health & Illness* 36, no. 6 (2014): 885–901. Accessed January 15, 2017. http://doi.org/10.1111/1467-9566.12122
49. Kirkman, Allison M. "Dementia in the News: The Media Coverage of Alzheimer's Disease". *Australasian Journal on Ageing* 25 (2006): 74–79.
50. Sontag, Susan. *La enfermedad y sus metáforas y El sida y sus metáforas* (Buenos Aires: Taurus, 2003), 16.
51. Sontag, Susan. *La enfermedad y sus metáforas y El sida y sus metáforas* (Buenos Aires: Taurus, 2003), 124.
52. Pardo, Rebeca. "Imágenes de la (des)memoria: narrativas visuales autorreferenciales del Alzheimer en Barcelona". Master Thesis, Universitat de Barcelona, 2014, p. 51. Accessed January 15, 2017. http://hdl.handle.net/2445/66651
53. Aznar Almazán, Yayo. *Insensatos: Sobre la representación de la locura* (Murcia: Editorial Micromegas, 2013), 57.
54. Mellby, Julie L. "Jean-Martin Charcot's Visual Psychology". *Graphic Arts Exhibitions, Acquisitions, and Other Highlights from the Graphic Arts Collection*, Blog of the Princeton University Library (07/24/2012). Accessed January 15, 2017. https://blogs.princeton.edu/graphicarts/2012/07/visual_psychology_and_jean-mar.html.

55. Hugh Welch Diamond was president of the Royal Photographic Society of London.
56. Nowadays, some applications use mobile phone cameras to detect or monitor certain illnesses.
57. Didi-Huberman, Georges. *La invención de la histeria: Charcot y la iconografía fotográfica de la Salpetriere* (Madrid: Cátedra, 2007).
58. Londe is listed as the "Director of the Photography Service at the Salpêtrière Hospice". His photography service was very important, for example, in constructing the psychiatric category of hysteria, using a large collection of images illustrating all periods and phases of the disease. Londe, Albert. *La Photographie médicale : application aux sciences médicales et physiologiques* (Paris: Gauthier-Villars et Fils, Imprimeurs-Libraires. Éditeurs de la Bibliothèque Photographique, 1893). Accessed January 15, 2017. http://cnum.cnam.fr/PDF/cnum_8KE360.pdf
59. Ristich De Groote, Michele. *La locura a través de los siglos* (Barcelona: Editorial Bruguera, 1970), 321
60. Translated from this quote in Spanish: "los síntomas exacerbados de la gran histeria de Charcot desaparecieron cuando los médicos dejaron de creer en ellos: existen formas de estar loco admitidas en cada cultura".
61. Huertas, Rafael. "Imágenes de la locura: El papel de la fotografía en la clínica psiquiátrica". In *Maneras de mirar. Lecturas antropológicas de la fotografía* vol. 1, Coord. By Carmen Ortiz, Cristina Sánchez-Carretero y Antonio Cea, 109–121. (Madrid: Consejo Superior de Investigaciones Científicas, 2005), 111.
62. Aznar Almazán, Yayo. *Insensatos: Sobre la representación de la locura* (Murcia: Editorial Micromegas, 2013), 57.
63. Moscoso, Javier. *Historia Cultural del dolor* (Madrid: Taurus, Santillana Ediciones Generales, 2011).
64. According to Oscar Martínez, some authors suggest that these photographs represent the origins of the deinstitutionalization movement for community mental health services and open hospitals. See Martínez, Oscar. "Periodistas y reporteros gráficos como agentes de cambio en psiquiatría. Imágenes denuncia para el recuerdo". *Revista de la Asociación Española de neuropsiquiatría* XXV, no. 96 (Oct./Dec. 2005), 15.
65. Huertas, Rafael. *Historia cultural de la psiquiatría: (Re)pensar la locura* (Madrid: Los Libros de la Catarata, 2012).
66. Foucault, Michel. *Historia de la locura en la época clásica II* (México, DF: Fondo de cultura económica, 2010); Foucault, Michel. *Historia de la*

locura en la época clásica I (México, DF: Fondo de cultura económica, 2011).
67. Goffman, Erving. *Internados. Ensayos sobre la situación social de los enfermos mentales* (Buenos Aires: Amorrortu, 2001).
68. Szasz, Thomas S. *El mito de la enfermedad mental* (Buenos Aires: Amorrortu Editores, 1994).
69. Depardon, Raymond. *Manicomio* (Paris: Fondation Cartier pour l'art contemporain, 2013).
70. Depardon, Raymond. *Manicomio* (Paris: Fondation Cartier pour l'art contemporain, 2013), 29 without numbers.
71. Martínez, Oscar, and Luisa Serrulla. "Siglo y medio de psiquiatría a través de la fotografía italiana". *FRENIA* VIII (2008): 183–206.
72. Poseck, Beatriz Vera. *Imágenes de la locura: la psicopatología en el cine* (Madrid: Calamar Ediciones, 2006).
73. Images available on the photographer's website: http://majadaniels.com/projects/into-oblivion/#PHOTO_39 (last seen, 26/12/2016).
74. Images available on the photographer's website: http://www.kennethohalloran.com/living-with-alzheimers/ (last seen, 26/12/2016).
75. Kirkman, Allison M. "Dementia in the News: The Media Coverage of Alzheimer's Disease". *Australasian Journal on Ageing* 25 (2006): 74.
76. Images available on the WPP website: http://www.worldpressphoto.org/collection/photo/2012/daily-life/alejandro-kirchuk (last seen, 26/12/2016).
77. Maragall, Pasqual, and Caro García. *Pasqual Maragall Mira* (Barcelona: Ed. Blume, 2010).
78. Pasqual Maragall was the 127th President of the Generalitat de Catalunya, the Mayor of Barcelona (1982 to 1997), and one of the authorities during the Barcelona Olympic Games (1992).
79. Pardo, Rebeca, and Montse Morcate. "Illness, Death and Grief: The Daily Experience of Viewing and Sharing Digital Images". In *Digital Photography and Everyday Life*, edited by Edgar Gómez Cruz and Asko Lehmuskallio (Routledge, 2016), 70–85.
80. Hirsch, Marianne. *FAMILY FRAMES. Photography, Narrative and Postmemory* (USA: Harvard University Press, 2002), 93.
81. Toledano, Phillip. *Days with My Father* (Auckland: PQ Blackwell Limited in association with Chronicle Books LLC, 2010).
82. Accessed May 5, 2015. http://www.dayswithmyfather.com/. No longer accessible online but the content is in the book by Toledano: *Days with My Father*.

83. Pardo, Rebeca, and Montse Morcate. "Illness, Death and Grief: The Daily Experience of Viewing and Sharing Digital Images". In *Digital Photography and Everyday Life*, edited by Edgar Gómez Cruz and Asko Lehmuskallio (Routledge, 2016), 70–85.
84. Accessed September 2, 2015. http://www.diariodeuncuidador.com/blog/
85. Accessed September 2, 2015. https://mividaconelalzheimer.wordpress.com
86. http://ellaelalzheimeryyo.blogspot.es/ (Last visited, 02/09/2015). The content of this blog has also been published as a book entitled *Vivir sin Vivir* (living without living) and some of the content is not available online at this moment.

Rebeca Pardo is a photographer and Professor of Photography at the Faculty of Arts, Universitat de Barcelona, and at the Faculty of Communication, Universitat Abat Oliba CEU, both of them in Barcelona, Spain. She is the Principal Investigator (PI) of the project "Sharing Pain and Grief Online" (http://deathandillness.com/). Her research and teaching interests include themes related to photography, illness, self-reference and visual narratives.

9

ADJOIN

Trish O'Shea, Mark Wilkinson, and Jackie Jones

TRISH: The Adjoin project involved us meeting on a regular basis and talking across a range of aspects of the disease of arthritis, why it happens and how we treat it. Through our discussions, exchange of experience, knowledge and understanding formed the focus, inspiration and content for ADJOIN. Often the discussions would be driven by my questioning in an attempt to understand Mark's work and to gain greater knowledge of the condition I live with. Mark gave me space, when needed, to share my experiences and feelings. Talking about arthritis and pain is often difficult, and I am thankful that he was very understanding when on a couple of occasions talking was hard for me. Mark shared his clinical experiences and the ongoing research he is involved in and his interest in patient participation. Adjoin therefore explores a developing narrative that was then interpreted and shared by me through using a variety of media such as photography, text, drawings and objects and is both factual

---

T. O'Shea (✉) • J. Jones
Sheffield, UK

M. Wilkinson
University of Sheffield, Sheffield, UK

and informative as well as autobiographical and personal. The intention is to share the resulting work with the public, with practitioners and with patients, in order to promote discussion about the condition of arthritis and its effects, and to promote the development of tools and techniques that could go towards enabling sufferers to communicate and share their experiences of the condition and of treatment, and thus help inform shared decision making in medical practice.

As part of Adjoin, I collaborated with photographer Jackie Jones. With Jackie's sensitive approach and patience I explored the physicality of how the experience of pain and restriction affects me. All the photographs presented here were taken by Jackie and, like the other visual pieces created along the way, are also a result of a two-way dialogue about my experiences and feelings and about my emotional reaction to having arthritis.

For the purpose of this chapter I have presented notes that I wrote as part of the project alongside and within the factual information. Some of the text is presented as in my notebooks, unedited, so as to present a real sense of the creative journey. I have recorded the dialogue between Mark and myself as a result of our meetings and that between Jackie and myself during our photographic sessions.

I am a visual artist who uses drawing, painting, text, the object, film and photography to present ideas and responses and often involve other people in many of the processes. I have experience in devising and delivering creative participatory projects, working with such themes as place, identity, culture, urban histories and the built environment. I have suffered from osteoarthritis most of my life, becoming more aware of the condition and the pain associated with it in my thirties. I am now fifty-six years old.

The artwork created for Adjoin was a result of a series of conversations with Professor Mark Wilkinson (orthopaedic surgeon and researcher). I started out on the project with some ideas about what additionally I would like to find out and understand about osteoarthritis in general and to share my own experiences of living with the condition. I'd like to thank Mark for being so generous with his time, and also very patient with me as I asked many questions! It has been a fascinating exchange and I feel privileged to have had the opportunity to do this work. The results have been a surprise to me—not only the physical pieces that have emerged, but also the emotional and psychological impact. To be able to make and create out of a "space" that for most of the time is a negative one (suffering from arthritis) has been very healing.

The balance between conveying facts and information along with my own personal experiences of the disease has been a challenge. I hope that within the work the viewer can gain knowledge about aspects of osteoarthritis and also about my experience of living with it and managing it. The work at times is open to interpretation. Within the context of the brief I have allowed myself to explore my own creativity. I would like to thank filmmaker and photographer Jackie Jones, who has been such a supporting presence, and has also produced beautiful work.

All work that I create sparks off connections, memories, associations and "Adjoin" has been no different. As I said to Mark one day, the showing of work is often the beginning of something rather than the end. I hope that because of the conversations with Mark and this creative process, ideas can be developed in order to support arthritis sufferers and promote active participation. There is no doubt that there are so many people within the medical world dedicated to helping, healing and finding ways to give relief to those who suffer from arthritis. I'd like to thank all those who continue with the work and those who have helped me personally.

Finally, I would like to dedicate this work to my parents, both arthritis sufferers, both strong and resilient and both helped, through joint replacements, to live full lives. Sadly, my father passed away on the 2nd August 2016 and my mother on the 17th December 2016.

Trish O'Shea 2017

* * *

It has been a delightful and inspiring experience working with Trish as the Adjoin project has developed. It has been a learning experience for both of us along the way. I have shared some of my learning experiences as a surgeon treating patients with arthritis, during our conversations. At the same time, I have learnt so much from Trish that has helped me better understand the human face of the disease.

Clinicians are generally confident in managing the care of patients suffering from arthritis. However, rarely do we have the opportunity to really get to know the person behind the disease, both their expectations and fears. I hope that in the bringing together of this project something of our shared-learning experience has been conveyed.

I have a particular interest in better understanding why some patients develop arthritis whilst others seem immune to its ravages. I am also interested in the workings of the shared decision-making process involved in agreeing individual treatment plans for patients. The exhibition material aims to display something of these insights into arthritis from both the patient's and the doctor's perspectives. It has been a very stimulating journey exploring these interests with Trish, and I am very grateful to her for sharing it with me.

Mark Wilkinson 2017

The beginning:

> *M*: "900,000 people in the UK suffer with arthritis, the cost to the economy each year is 14 billion pounds. The cost to the NHS is 5 billion pounds. It is the fourth biggest cost for the NHS in England and Wales. 20% of over 45's and 40% of over 70's have knee arthritis symptoms".

I wrote these statistics down as Mark spoke. I had to re-read the words a few times in order to grasp the enormity of them and what it meant. I thought that's an awful lot of money and an awful lot of suffering. That's a mountain of pain and discomfort. But where are all these people? I started to collect the empty paracetamol packets.

> *T*: "It's interesting how people don't really talk openly about arthritis. It doesn't seem to be I the public domain as with other diseases".
>
> *M*: "Arthritis doesn't kill people. It doesn't therefore seem a priority".
>
> *T*: "But it kills a way of life?"
>
> *M*: "Oh yes. It is the hidden disease".
>
> *T*: "That's a lot of people suffering in silence".
>
> *M*: "Yes".
>
> *T*: "I think being able to talk about the condition, how it affects you, makes you feel is really important. Being able to talk about the pain and discomfort is crucial, to externalise it and share it. I think that it is important as part of a sufferer's treatment. Do you agree?"
>
> *M*: "Absolutely. The NHS is generally good at managing diseases, but there is also a person suffering the condition. The NHS provides space for patient education about their condition, but, given the rush to deal with

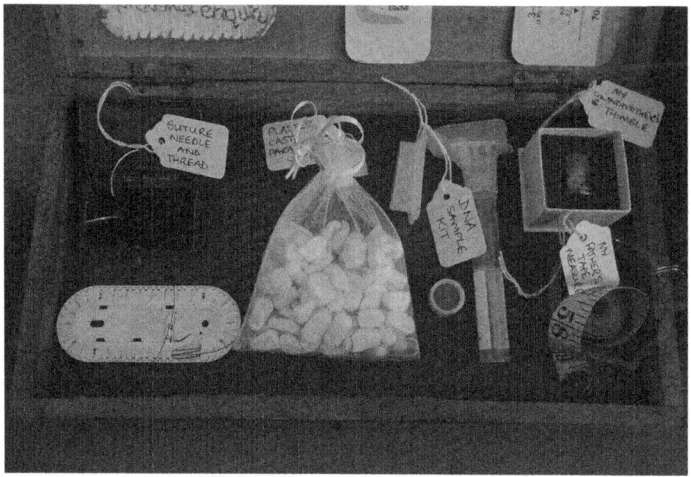

Fig. 9.1 Collection by Trish O'Shea

the treatment, patients can feel that the personalised element of their care is left behind. Other organisations, such as Arthritis Care UK, provide a forum to help fill some of this space, and promoting the opportunity for patients, their friends, family and carers to share their experiences".

Only relatively recently have I been able to talk about my arthritis and how the pain affects me on a daily basis. I found to begin with that talking about it was a very emotional experience and made me cry. I'm not alone in that. Like anything that hurts you, or makes life difficult, that is tiring and draining—arthritis engenders deep emotions. These emotions are often "kept in" in order to continue. When talked about, it is only natural to reveal sadness, anger, frustration and hence the tears. I accept that part of the condition now and understand it is important to talk. Acceptance of a lot of stuff around arthritis helps reduce the pain one suffers. I cried at times when I spoke with Mark and he understood, and gave me time.

M: "There are 100,000 knee replacement operations each year for knee arthritis in England and Wales alone. The great majority (80% of patients) are very pleased with the outcome from their knee replacement surgery".
T: "Can the 80% and the remaining 20% be analysed in terms of the age of the patients? Are most of the 80% elderly? What is 'young' in terms

of the age of people who undergo knee replacement surgery? Does age have a real affect upon outcome?"

M: "Younger patients are more likely to be dissatisfied, but this is not a strict rule. I would say younger than 40 years of age is young for knee replacement. There is an effect with age, with younger patients wearing the knee out earlier".

M: "I have a specific interest in arthritis research and how it may run in families. About 50% of our risk for getting arthritis is due to our lifestyle and 50% we inherit from our parents".

T: "What is meant by environment?"

M: "Age, sex, occupation, previous injury/damage, everything that isn't in your DNA"

T: "Is there a gender difference?"

M: "About 60% of knee OA occurs in women and 40% in men"

I am too young to have had a knee replacement—surely? I am too young to have all this pain surely? I was once talking with a friend about the work involved in living with arthritis. We talked about pain. My friend could not, just could not, imagine living most days and often nights in pain. I said that I could not imagine living without pain. Pain has redefined me. Pain separates me.

Walkingswimming gardening dancing sitting standing lying down getting up bending turning sleeping making reaching stepping.

LET'S TRY to go up the stairs, go down the stairs, catch the bus, get into the taxi, get out of the taxi, sit on the floor, get up, walk up the hill, go down the hill, sit down, get up, get over the stile, turn over in bed, swim, get into the car, get out of the car, get up when a goal is scored, dig the earth, stand, reach down to the cupboard, wait.... Let's not.

Mark: "Lots and lots of genes contribute to the condition of osteoarthritis, but we need to understand the whole picture in order to progress towards developing treatments that will change the experience of patients with osteoarthritis. Using the analogy of the haystack and needles we need more 'hay' in order to find the relevant needles. We need a lot more people from whom we can collect DNA".

When Mark mentioned haystacks, I thought of Monet's haystacks. All golden and rich in deep colour—warm, dense, soft, round, still, hazy and vivid. Then I remembered me as a child on my friend's farm clambering for hours over hay and jumping and rolling and laughing. I remembered evenings in the summer sun, feeling the dying heat on my skin and bones and the suppleness of my young body shifting and moving in between and over the straw bales that would become the haystack. I thought about running and how I have been unable to run in a long while now. No more running for buses now. I sometimes struggle to walk at a good pace now.

Mark: "Research is like 'finding signals' in all the noise".

Trying to understand the genetics of arthritis is difficult when it all seems so complex, but there is an enigmatic beauty within the language—deep, deep mystery. To realise that so much time, effort and money is going into trying to find the cause of arthritis is humbling. The fact that the causes of arthritis are still somewhat of a mystery is challenging and sad. But great things are being achieved and discovered.

How might I depict this language? How might I present the facts and enable the viewer to understand and appreciate them? I remember my Mum trying to teach me to knit and sew. The idea of the stitched line kept emerging. It seemed to link to the genetic theme and the skills of the Mother being passed on, as well as the disease of the parents being passed on. The stitched line evoked the very real experience of being stitched up, and the resulting line in the flesh and made me think of the surgeon as textile artist and sculptor. So, I began to embroider letters, words and numbers.

Chromosome 3 with rS6976 embroidered onto support bandage fabric.

Chromosome 9 close to ASTN2 embroidered onto one of my Mother's bandages.

Chromosome 12 close to CHST 11, FTO gene, embroidered within a circle of chain stitch.

I asked Mark to stitch just so I could watch him use the surgeon's needle and thread. I gave him two pieces of elastic support bandage to join.

Mark: "There is no medication that can stop the progression of osteoarthritis. The best treatment at present is joint replacement. I hope through research we find a cure, and that advances in the understanding of the disease means surgeons become redundant".

Joint replacement is truly a remarkable process giving sufferers new life and hope. Arthritis can feel like a hopeless disease. It can create a real sense of loss. It is a physical, emotional and psychological disease and the core of it is the pain. Living with arthritis takes great strength and great physical and mental fortitude. Sufferers require encouragement, tenderness and love as well as sometimes a combat-like stance—a "never give up" attitude.

I made "Tower of Strength" which was all the empty paracetamol packets on top of one another, glued one by one and tied tight. On top of the tower stood a tiny figure covered in melted wax. I drew the packets creating detailed pencil studies. I like to ask people to really look at the seemingly mundane and ordinary.

> M: "Pain is a dominant feature of arthritis, and physical restriction is also a symptom. Arthritis is a real burden and can cause decades of personal disability. The emotional response to the pain of arthritis is very variable. In some people it can be an ignoring, whilst in others it can be a catastrophising response. This sort of pain response has proven to be a difficult element of knee replacements".
>
> T: "Why? In what way?"
>
> M: "Central pain sensitisation is a fairly common problem that causes pain persistence in some patients, like phantom limb pain in some amputees. Pain catastrophisation is a rare problem, but it is useful to be aware of in patients with chronic pain sensitisation as it indicates a psychological dimension to the problem. When one suffers from chronic pain it becomes hard wired and persists. Touch can be a stimulus—even the lightest of touch can be painful".

"So is that why my legs are so sensitive and painful to touch? The slightest knock or pressure is so painful at times it literally makes me wince. When did this happen? Is there a cure?"

I made small figures using wax, bandage and pins. It was good to be able to twist the shapes and therefore present an idea of discomfort.

> M: "Hyper-sensitivity is one feature of 'central pain sensitisation' and is how the stimulus from the knee is interpreted in the central nervous system. This is when the brain interprets the stimulus as a 'danger'

signal and a reaction to a noxious stimulus. Consequently, wearing trousers, having the weight of bed covers or the lightest touch can be uncomfortable. This involves skin and tissues and is a feature of chronic pain".

T: "But we all experience pain so differently and we all have different ways of describing, measuring, assessing pain? It is a very personal experience".

M: "Yes, it is difficult—different people describe pain in different ways, and some people have a greater reaction to pain than others. Some people might even describe pain in terms of colours and odours".

On a scale from one to ten, how would you assess your pain **now**, at this moment?

| 1 | 2 | 3 | 4 | 5 | 6 | 7 | 8 | 9 | 10 |

If you could draw lines to depict your pain and how it changes, what lines would you draw I wonder?

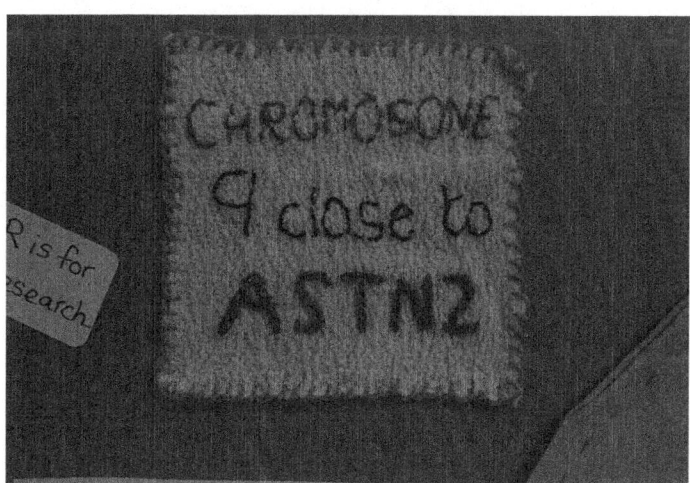

Fig. 9.2 Sample by Trish O'Shea

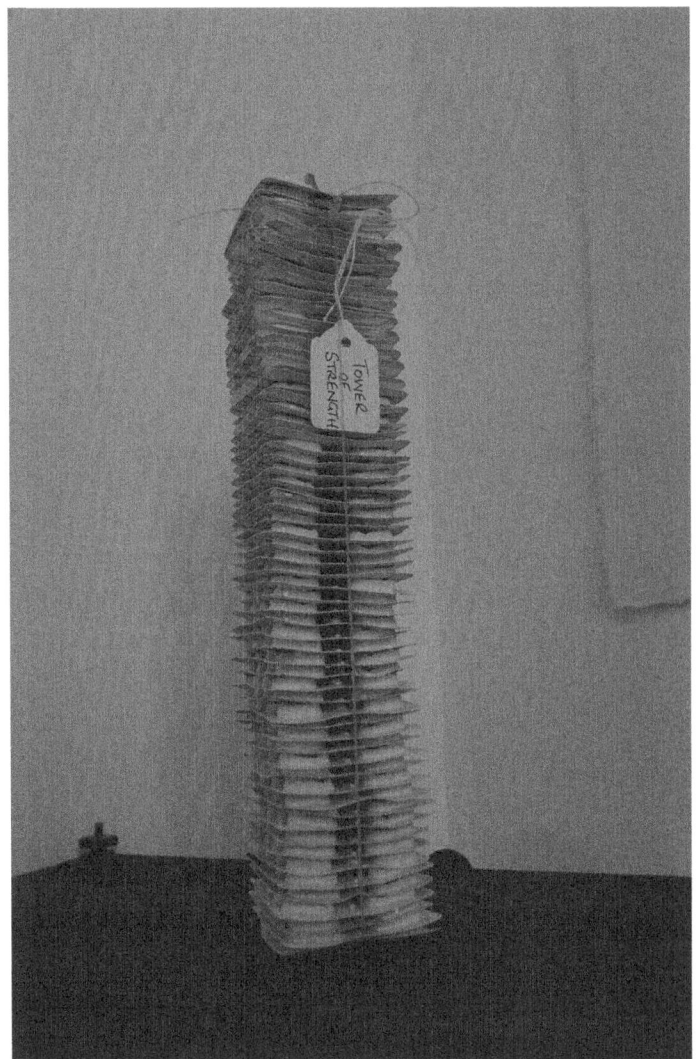

Fig. 9.3 Tower of strength by Trish O'Shea

How can I depict the pain management? How can I show how pain varies from one day to the next? That pain is a response to a range of activities and is not static. I decided to include a standard figure shape from a hospital information sheet. I recreated the figure in stitched line, monoprint, collage cut-out and incorporated text.

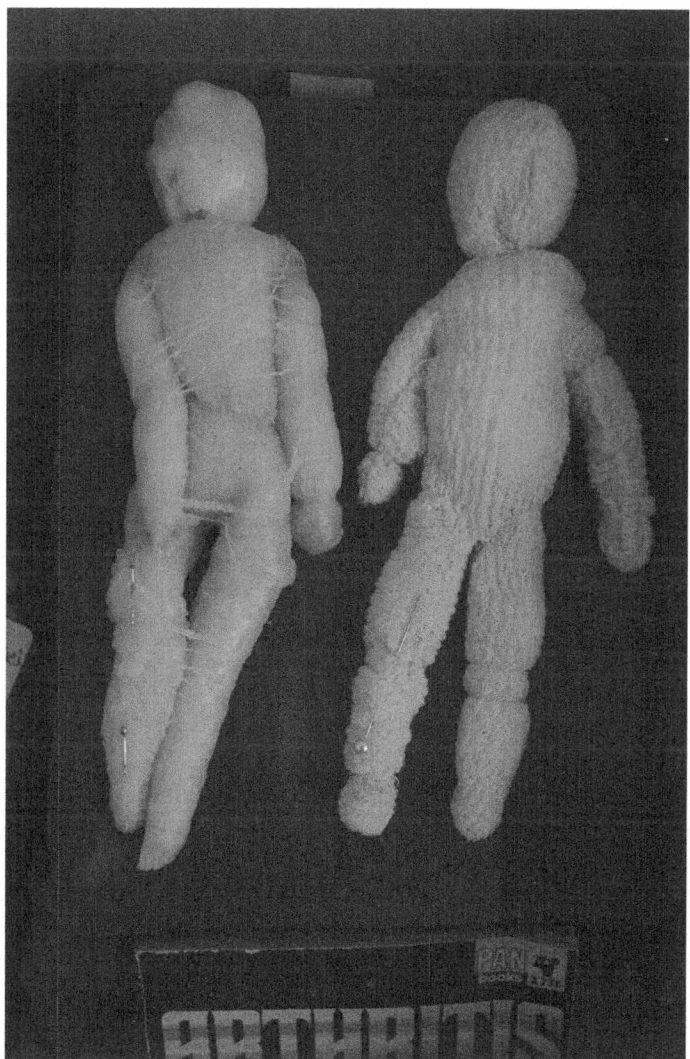

Fig. 9.4 Restriction by Trish O'Shea

Making plans can be difficult. Staying positive is an ongoing challenge. Constant management is essential. Planning ahead. Preparation (both physical and mental) is often needed in order to get the most out of events and activities.

REST- EXERCISE- DIET- ACTIVITY- REST- DIET- EXERCISE – REST

I love to be in water. Gliding. Weightless. Cool against the skin. Water is the place where I feel strong. My muscles released from the tightness. I still do hydrotherapy exercises. I like to float on my back. I love the heat of the sauna reaching deep into my bones.

Osteo - (prefix): Combining form meaning bone. From the Greek "osteon", bone.

Pain = Tears, Fatigue, Anger, Fear, Frustration.
Tears, Fatigue, Anger, Fear, Frustration = Pain.
Exercise = A sense of achievement, progress, hope. Break the cycle.

Be careful not to do too much exercise. Know your body. Know when to stop. Balanced diet, balanced exercise, balanced rest, balanced activity… see-saw.
Phenotype: the physical characteristics of something living, especially those characteristics that can be measured.

M: "Bio markers: an individual's response to pain may be influenced by measurable biomarkers".
T: "Is this a genetic factor? What is a biomarker?"
M: "A biomarker is any blood, urine or other test that can be done to diagnose a condition or predict response to treatment. It can be genetic, or any other thing that has predictive or diagnostic value. There are no established biomarkers for osteoarthritis".
T: "No biomarkers for arthritis?"
M: "No".
T: "Really?"
M: "No".
T: "Oh!"
M: "Despite extensive efforts, we have found only a few of the inherited risk factors for osteoarthritis, despite knowing that it accounts for 50% of our risk of getting the disease".

What genes cause arthritis?
How can more DNA be collected?
Are you looking in the right haystacks?

Doing things I really enjoy helps and "being in the moment" and I love walking in nature. Despite the occasional challenges of terrain, being in nature is healing. Recording nature through photography or through drawing and painting enables me to connect with something other than myself, other than my physical state. Being in nature is healing both physically and psychologically, and I think it should be prescribed.

See over there where I saw the two deer…

Genotype: the particular type and arrangement of genes that each organism has. The genotype is the part (DNA sequence) of the genetic makeup of a cell, and therefore of an organism or individual, which determines a specific characteristic (phenotype) of that cell/organism/individual.

Heterogeneity is a word that signifies diversity. A classroom consisting of people from lots of different backgrounds would be considered having the quality of heterogeneity. The prefix "hetero-" means "other or different", while the prefix "homo-" means "the same".

Genome: the complete set of genetic material of a human, animal, plant, or other living thing.

On a scale from one to ten, how would you assess how beautiful you are, at this moment?

1	2	3	4	5	6	7	8	9	10

I love birdwatching. Being still and silent is a wonderfully healing experience. Engaging with that which is outside of you detracts from the pain and discomfort.

Although gardening is getting more and more difficult, I endeavour to keep doing it. Going slower, taking time, resting, managing expectations, being realistic, asking for help. There is nothing more satisfying than slowly and carefully digging up your own potatoes. Or watching someone else do it for you. And then a robin comes close.…

gardening growing making baking
reading walking swimming slow dancing
friendship family Sheffield Wednesday
creativity film nature art music

aetiopathogenesis: the cause and development of a disease, especially within cells
"aetio-" The Greek root for "cause", as in aetiology.
…. finding signals in all the noise. Listen to that birdsong, it's beautiful. Everything has to be done slower. Be careful.

Me: "Why am I doing this project? I must be mad".
Friend: "Because you need to?" *Me*: "I'm not sure what the point is at the moment. I'm worried it will all seem negative and without hope".
Friend: "Life and Art can be like that".
Me: "I know. I'm in a process of searching for some understanding and how to respond. I feel like I have to give greater understanding and insight and give answers. How am I going to make Art out of all this?"
Friend: "Come on, you know by now that Art often creates more mystery and asks more questions than it answers. That's the wonderful thing about it!"
Me: "That's so interesting, Mark said that about the research he does".

Accepting the condition and trying not to let fear take over is the challenge and ongoing aim. Knowing that it is likely that the condition will get worse

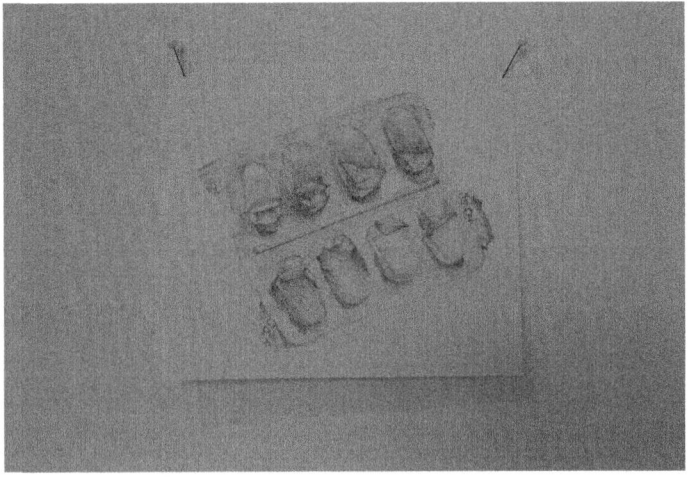

Fig. 9.5 Pain relief by Trish O'Shea

as time passes can be frightening and worrying. Trying to avoid thinking "It's not fair". Celebrate all that is good in life as much as possible. Push yourself to do things. But also allow yourself time and space to feel what you feel, and recognise those feelings. Talking about how you feel is healing.

On a scale from one to ten, how would you assess your self-confidence **now**, at this moment?

1	2	3	4	5	6	7	8	9	10

I made a list of all the health practitioners who had helped me to heal, fifteen different disciplines. Many individuals. I stitched their roles onto a support stocking.

love yourself   *you are beautiful.*

"CONFIDENTIAL" *Progress Reports 2010*—a collaborative piece by photographer Jackie Jones and visual artist Trish O'Shea

"CONFIDENTIAL" is a result of conversations between Jackie and myself about me living with osteoarthritis and the pain and restriction it causes. Conversations continued about hospital visits over a period of years and being examined, studied, x-rayed and questioned. The difficult and rather frightening decision to have a knee replacement, then the extreme pain of the treatment and long recovery, which brings about a "renaissance" of sorts. Text from x-ray reports was transferred onto opaque paper and the paper attached to clip files over the photographs. The photographs of me were thus partly hidden and could only be seen as a "hazy" presence. To see the photographs properly the viewer had to lift the paper and look under. The colours of the cloth (and I realised only later a lot of the shapes and forms I created with my body) were inspired by renaissance art. I really wanted to show people what the pain can feel like, but was challenged as to how and why?

I was aware that Trish had arthritis, but until I worked with her on the project I had no idea how debilitating or common it was. The brief was to explore how we could visualise and document what arthritis felt like through photography. As the project progressed, my understanding of the disease grew enormously, but I had no idea how we were going to visualise it in a way that would interest the general public. In the discussions we had once we got the go-ahead, I showed her photographs that I liked and thought had some potential. Some of them were images of women in unusual poses and some were photographs that looked like paintings.

Trish wanted to be the subject of the photos so we took the plunge and did a shoot in her small attic room. Trish bandaged up her legs, and used other health aids that she was encouraged to use to make herself feel better. I was fairly happy with the results, but Trish was unsure about her head being visible. A while later we arranged the second shoot. Clearly agitated, Trish said, 'This is going to be a performance piece', and lay down on the floor, and tried out different ideas, including using charcoal to draw on her legs.

I was stood raised above her, grabbing shots as she expressed how she was feeling. She had brought some beautiful blue material and wrapped herself up in it. Out of that shoot, one image captured our imagination. It was Trish wrapped in material that was trailing behind her, her head covered and her arms wrapped around herself. It looked like a painting, and although she didn't look happy, it looked beautiful.

Around this time Trish sent me her x-ray reports from over the last few years. I was fascinated by the language, and began extracting phrases and sentences, none of which I understood. For the third and final shoot, we went and bought several pieces of different coloured material. Some of these were laid on the floor, and some were wrapped around Trish. I shot dozens of images and afterward we went through them. I then edited the ones we were both pleased with, ending up with 16 distinct A4 size images.

The next problem we had to solve was how to display the text from the consultant with the photos. We both had the same idea of using tissue paper with the text on it, covering the photos, which were then fixed on to clipboards evoking what would be seen on the end of a hospital bed. To view the photos, you had to lift the tissue paper invoking a sense of prying. The end result showed a great deal about Trish as a living breathing human being, battling with a painful debilitating condition. The clinical language written on the paper covering her, which was purely concerned with the physical progression of the disease, provided a stark contrast to the images. In the end, we are much more than physical beings, and I think the photography and Trish's other exhibits illustrated that idea well. (Jackie Jones)

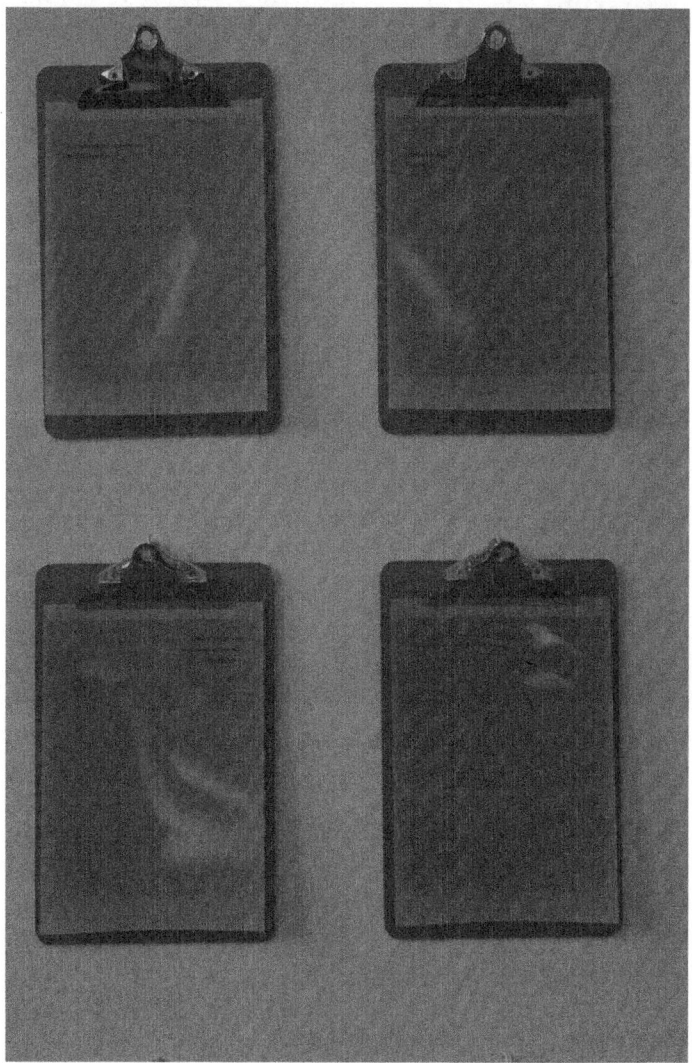

Fig. 9.6 Confidential, by Trish O'Shea and Jackie Jones

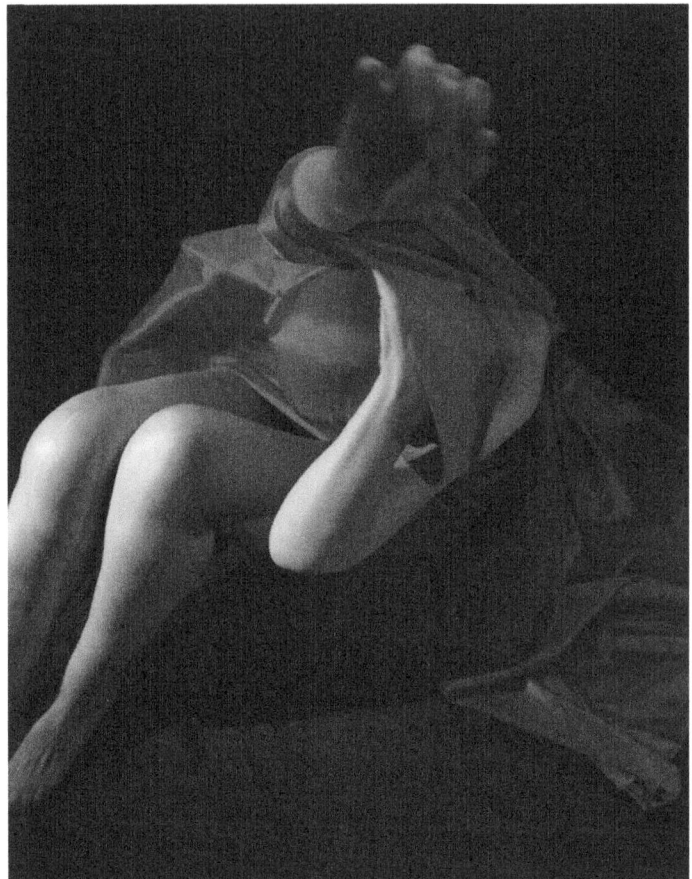

Fig. 9.7 Detail of confidential by Trish O'Shea and Jackie Jones

The images explore and depict the desire to escape, to float, to be transformed and to be physically represented as fluid and supple, when the reality is different. The cloth hides my body—reflecting my self-consciousness when it comes to my body being viewed. The clinical language describes me and reveals the gradual deterioration of bone and joint.

26/8/10 8.44am Radiology XR Right knee
There is marked narrowing of the right patella femoral joint. There is oesteophytic lipping and early narrowing of the medial compartments of both knees. There is possible loose body in the right supra-patella pouch.

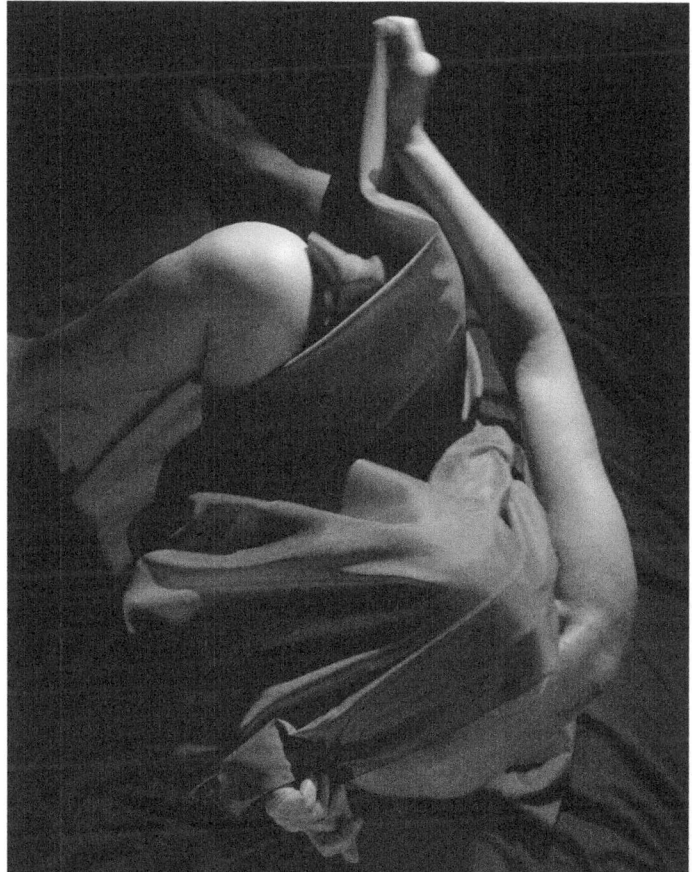

Fig. 9.8 Detail of confidential, by Trish O'Shea and Jackie Jones

At first I wanted to just try and shock people into looking at how the pain sometimes feels. I thought I might wrap barbed wire around my knees. But that would have been too literal and would have hindered questioning from the viewer.

16/8/11 9.59 Radiology XR Right knee
   Tricompartmental osteoarthritis. Particularly severe, affecting the patellofemoral joint. Similar less severe appearances on the left.

I was worried about being too intimate, showing too much. I have an ambivalent relationship with my body. We tried things. I wrapped lengths of

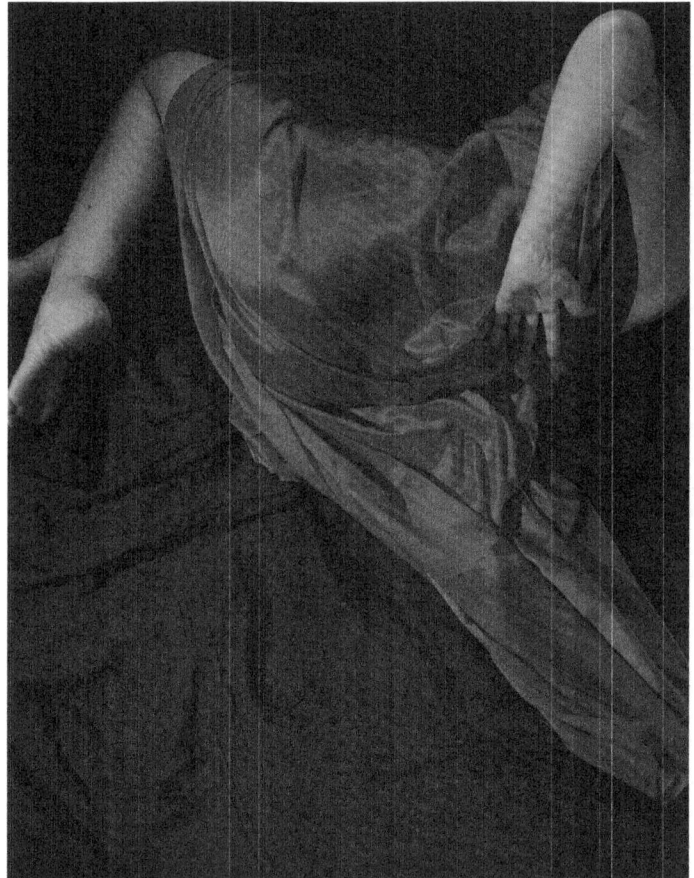

Fig. 9.9 Detail of confidential by Trish O'Shea and Jackie Jones

bandages around my knees. Binding them in order to show the sense of tightness and restriction. I found this a very therapeutic act. Jackie photographed my scarring and my swollen joints.

13/12/12 14.54 Radiology XR Both knees.
There is marked narrowing of the patellofemoral joints. There is prominent osteophytic lipping of the main compartments, more marked medially with early narrowing of the medial compartment of the left knee.

Gradually through trying things out and talking through the process it became clear to me that as well as wanting to show the pain I also wanted to show a sense of innerness. A sense of the pain within that is often masked. I also didn't want to "shock". I wanted to create something beguiling, mysterious and dynamic—like a visual analogy of the clinical language used to describe the condition and the process of degeneration.

31/5/13 10.31 Radiology MRI right knee
There is complete loss of the patellofemoral articular cartilage. There is marked narrowing of the patellofemoral joint space with subchondral marrow oedema in both patella and the trochlear. There is a joint effusion. There is a large multilocular cyst anteromedial to the knee joint. Cruciate ligaments appear intact. The menisci and MCL appear intact. There is thinning of the articular cartilage in the lateral compartment with prominent oesteophytic lipping.

We began to play with the language and the images. I looked to Renaissance Art and the theme "re-birth" for colour, shape and form. Using brightly coloured fabric and (with difficulty) pushing my body into contorted shapes beneath the fabric we began a process of searching for the visual language to show the sense of being trapped, for the need to escape and a sense of an inner and hidden world, of distress masked. And yet, we wanted the images to also depict a sense of mystery, of strength and of beauty.

14/4/14 16.27 Radiology XR right knee
There is marked narrowing of the patellofemoral joint, there is prominent osteophytic lipping of the main compartments with early narrowing of the medial compartment.

It was Jackie who came up with the idea of printing the text from the x-ray results onto opaque paper and placing the paper over the photographs, thus hiding the image and inviting the viewer to lift the paper to view the photograph beneath and to "peer" at the image—or not.

1/7/14 17.00 Radiology XR right knee
Right total knee replacement. There are locules of gas within the subcutaneous tissues.

The process of producing the photographs was a healing process in itself, a time to talk openly about the condition and the effect upon the body as a whole. I became more in touch with my physicality as I moved and stretched and talked.

    24/4/15 16.11 Radiology XR right knee. Right knee TKR. No complication shown.
        Lethargy post TKA. ? Vit D def? TFT abnormality

…. finding signals in all the noise

Trish O'Shea is a visual artist, creative engagement practitioner and educator who utilises drawing, painting, text, print, the object and photography to present her ideas and responses. Trish is experienced in devising and delivering creative participatory projects. Themes such as place, identity, histories are often an inspiration. As well as developing her own personal work, Trish often involves and works creatively with individuals and groups in many of her processes, in order for experiences to be shared and revealed.

Mark Wilkinson is Professor of Orthopaedics at the University of Sheffield, and an honorary consultant orthopaedic surgeon at Sheffield Teaching Hospitals NHS Foundation Trust. Mark's clinical work focuses on the treatment of arthritis. His research work is aimed at helping us better understand what causes arthritis, and how people respond differently to the disease. He is also interested in developing decision aids to help patients make more informed choices about their treatment options when facing the disease.

Jackie Jones is an accomplished video producer, TV lighting-camera operator and photographer, and as a video producer she has worked on many educational and training products, and also national productions happening locally. She has worked extensively as an educator, but producing images for her own purposes and others has been a life-long passion.

10

Face2face: Sharing the Photograph Within Medical Pain Encounters—A Means of Democratisation

Deborah Padfield and Joanna M. Zakrzewska

The Challenge of Pain to Communication

Pain is common and difficult to communicate,[1,2,3] or reduce into the verbal or numerical scales commonly used in clinical practice. Academics from Scarry[4] to Charon[5] have argued that pain resists description in language, while Biro[6] and Bourke[7] have argued conversely that it generates language. This paper identifies the limitations of verbal language and current standardised scores for assessing pain, arguing instead that visual images (in particular the photograph) can elicit language and narrative capable of expanding and improving communication and clinician-patient interaction specifically within medical pain consultations, but with implications for use in other contexts.

The paper focuses on a collaborative photographic project between Fine Art and Medicine, *face2face*,[8,9,10] at a leading London teaching

---

D. Padfield (✉)
Slade School of Fine Art, University College, London

J.M. Zakrzewska
Eastman Dental Hospital and Pain Management Centre, University College London Hospitals, NHS Foundation Trust, London, UK

hospital, itself building on an earlier sciart project, *perceptions of pain*.[11,12] Both projects sought to develop a visual as opposed to verbal language as an alternative vehicle for communicating and capturing pain. Contrary to expectation it became possible to hypothesise that the images' most powerful potential was not in replacing verbal language but in regenerating it, catalysing new descriptors for pain from sufferers' own worlds (as opposed to the pre-prescribed words of the McGill Pain Questionnaire), and highlighting the most problematic aspects of their lived experience. The method of using visual images as a communication aid[12] is proposed as a complement rather than an alternative to existing measures, building on methods of photo-elicitation in the social sciences and the current growing interest in narrative medicine and the influence of the arts and humanities on medical practice. The study builds on calls for the democratisation of medicine, arguing that the '*humanities educate for democratic habits and … medicine is in need of democratization, bearing a historical legacy of authority-led structures and hierarchical teamwork*'.[13]

Redefining Chronic Pain

American physician and academic David Biro argues for a redefinition of pain to one which makes no distinction between emotional and physical pain.[14] In this context images are useful, able to collapse both within a single image. The photograph's ability to signify multiple meanings refutes reductionist readings along Cartesian binaries, opening up discussions around interpretation, significance and meaning. Biro proposes the International Association for the Study of Pain (IASP's) definition be expanded to include '*the aversive feeling of injury to one's person and the threat of further potentially more serious injury. It can be described metaphorically*'.[15] He argues this would reduce semantic confusion around pain, and provide a better framework for managing patients, encouraging new ways of treating them by removing a distinction between actual and perceived damage, between physical and emotional pain. Patients' perception of their pain and the narrative into which they fit it thereby becomes central to the discussion of pain.[2] Images can be a way of revealing this framework and the significance of pain experience for an individual. Bourke[7,16] argues that pain is experienced culturally and socially. Images may be a powerful tool for eliciting the context in which pain is experienced by an individual and unravelling its meaning with them.

With no biomarkers, pain remains a subjective sensation relying on the patient's story and on the sufferer being able to express it.[17] As Boddice argues, those with pain reach not only to express it linguistically but bodily, orally and emotionally.[18] It is unlikely that medical imaging devices will ever be able to interpret or communicate this complex integration of corporeal and emotional experience we call pain. We are therefore reliant on a mutually trusting rapport between clinician and patient to create an environment in which effective two-way communication can take place.

Medical Anthropologist Arthur Kleinman argues for the value of integrating *'physiological, psychological and social meanings'* of pain and illness.[19,20,21] Narrative medicine is one means of achieving this, as it *'allows the patient to be heard, begin healing, and may be just what we need to reduce the unequal burden of pain and improve the quality of pain care for all'*.[22] Academic and physician Rita Charon, who coined the term narrative medicine, claims that *'one of the central aspects of pain medicine that is undetectably central to all of medicine is narrative'*[23] observing that *'built into the very nature of narrative is that it is shared'*.[24] It is in this context that images are proposed as a potential means of eliciting and sharing the narrative necessary for healing—in its broadest sense.

Use of Photographic Images as a Tool for Eliciting Pain Narratives

There has been a growing interest in the use of images, and in particular photographic images, to elicit narrative from those affected by trauma, illness or pain. Harrison's review of the use of visual methodologies in the social sciences starts from a premise that the visual has been, *'until recently, a neglected dimension in our understanding of social life, despite the role of vision in other disciplines'*.[25] This is changing, and from as far back as artist and activist Jo Spence[26,27,28] to more recent projects such as those of Alan Radley,[29,30,31,32] Sara Bro[33] and Johanna Willenfelt[34] to current collectives such as Collen's Pain Exhibit,[35,36] the work of Pat Walton exploring the everyday life of families living with chronic pain and its impact on interfamilial relationships, Susanne Main's work exploring the value of online exhibitions[37] and the Flickr and Tumblr sites examined recently by Gonzalez-Polledo and Tarr,[38] photographs are being used as vehicles through which those who are ill or in pain can communicate their experience to others, and through which they can seek to understand it themselves. In the face of often invisible and intangible experience, pain sufferers have also turned to metaphor[6,14] as well as images,[39] and frequently to both. There is an innate urge to translate the private, invisible experience of pain into something tangible and visible to others, and both metaphor and visual images are a means of doing this.

Other projects have also capitalised on the need for a visual representation of pain asking patients to draw their experience.[40,41,42] The Pain T project set up by pain specialist, Dr Dietmar Harmann, ran a series of art workshops in conjunction with art therapists, where those with pain were invited to draw or paint their experience.[43] There has been a burgeoning of projects exploring digital means of representing pain visually such as McMahon's web-based Iconic Pain Assessment Tool—IPAT[44,45] and Stones' research into the value of picture-led tools for pain management.[46] Closs et al.[47] have recently attempted to test twelve images '*depicting sensory qualities*' of pain for their use in differentiating between neuropathic and nociceptive pain. There is, however, an inbuilt problematic in assessing images for their 'accuracy', as it could be argued that one of the characteristics of images is their openness to different interpretations and that there is no such thing as an 'accurate' or universal image.

Main argues that creative methods can be used to communicate the experience of living with chronic pain when expression through language fails.[37] Many film-makers and performance artists have offered insights into the experience of living with chronic illness and pain, for example Stephen Dwoskin (*Pain is …* and *intoxicated by my own illness*), Bob Flanagan, Martin O' Brien, and Laura Dannequin's performance work based on her personal experience of living with chronic pain.[48] There is thus a trend towards making visual shareable representations of pain and illness, which are outside the body.[61]

Reasons for Investigating Images as an Alternative Language with Which to Communicate or Share Pain Experience

Limitations of Current Medical Measures and Need for An Alternative Measure for Evaluating Pain

Most current medical pain measures commonly provide pre-existing verbal or numerical scales/lists to select from such as the verbal rating scale, visual analogue scales, Brief Pain Inventory and the McGill Pain Questionnaire (MPQ). These can fail to capture experience as complex and multifaceted as pain, as well as failing to provide opportunities for patients to generate their own language. The MPQ asks patients to constrict their experience into pre-existing formulae, a list of 78 different adjectives. It thus denies people with pain an opportunity to create their own metaphors using language drawn from their own social worlds. It is in the struggle to find apposite words, to create new descriptors that more unusual and individually significant words emerge. The subtitle of Scarry's seminal tome[4] references the making and the unmaking of the world following pain. A re-making of the world following pain happens largely through language; it is vital that this language is drawn from sufferers' own worlds—and photographs are one means of generating such language.

Impact of Inadequate Means of Expressing or Measuring Pain

Pain experiences are not easy to fit within the existing reductive measures or frameworks into which the medical system tries to place them, such as the Numerical Rating Scale (rate your pain on a scale of 1 to 10). This serves to increase the isolation of sufferers—in turn affecting pain experience itself.[49] There is now considerable evidence that pain and emotional processing systems interact.[50,51,52,53,54] It follows that discussion of the emotional impact and/or components of pain could not only reduce isolation but be pivotal to healing. If photographic images can catalyse patients' own language, it should be easier for those witnessing pain to enter the worlds in which that pain is happening, share the burden of pain and discuss mutually agreeable treatment plans more fruitfully.

Face2face 2008–2013

Overview of the *Face2face* Photographic Project, 2008–2013

The project had several strands: art workshops for clinicians and patients to attend together; the co-creation of photographs with facial pain patients before, during and after treatment, making visible and re-enforcing changes patients had made in the perception of their pain; the creation of an image resource integrating photographs from both *Perceptions of Pain* and *face2face* as an innovative communication tool for clinical use; a study piloting the image resource as a pack of 54 PAIN CARDS in pain consultations,[10] and an artist's film focusing on doctor-patient dialogue and the role of narrative, positively reviewed in the medical and general press.[55]

In contrast to *Perceptions of Pain*, face2face focused mainly on facial pain. Facial pain has all the difficulties associated with musculo-skeletal pain, as well as additional ones specific to the face. The canvas most of us use to express pain is the face, and yet when that canvas is itself in pain, it is difficult to express in a way which others can read accurately.

Face2face: Research Questions

Initially the overall research question we asked was:

> Could a visual language provide an alternative means for communicating pain?

During the research and analyses we developed a more nuanced approach, asking:

Can, and if so, how can photographs of pain placed between clinician and patient improve dialogue and rapport in medical pain consultations? Can photographs generate an expanded and richer vocabulary capable of bridging the space between the person in pain and the person witnessing/treating it? Can photographic images re-balance the patient-clinician encounter and improve the quality of communication and interaction in the consulting room?

Aims and Methodology

A key aim of co-creating images of pain with sufferers was to make pain visible and shareable with the hope of improving mutual understanding between those witnessing and those experiencing pain. Individual workshops aimed to co-create images which, as closely as possible, represented the pain sufferers' unique experience of pain. The sessions (numbering between nine and twelve) happened at three points during their treatment journey; before, during or after management/treatment in order to prevent those with pain from being trapped not just within their pain but within a single negative image. By working with people with pain at different points in their management journey, we were able to produce a collection of images reflecting a broad range of intensities and pain qualities. This arc of time allowed the images to represent changes sufferers had made in their perception of pain and to reflect a sense of movement and transformation where present. Working at different points in the management journey was a way of addressing the sense of stasis and paralysis so often accompanying the language and experience of chronic pain states, as well as a means of eliciting pertinent narrative and significant emotion to surface to be discussed.

The basic method of co-creating images with pain sufferers has been reported fully in several publications,[10,11] but a brief summary follows.

Face2face: Sessions Co-creating the Photographs

The bulk of the creative practice of the *face2face* project involved co-creating portraits or images of their pain with five pain patients from UCLH with different types of facial pain. During *Perceptions of Pain*, I had developed a process of co-creating images with pain patients, which aimed to give visual form to each person's unique experience of pain. Combining the creativity and strengths of pain sufferer and artist enables us to arrive together at a stronger series of images than either I or they would have arrived at alone, able to resonate with people outside the process. Patients who co-create images directly control how their pain is visualised and represented to others rather than being placed on the receiving end of the medical gaze.

The sessions were individual, mostly in rooms booked in the hospital, but occasionally at other significant locations chosen by participants, for example walking round London looking for derelict buildings or in a participant's garden in West Hampstead. All sessions were audio-recorded and later transcribed. They numbered between nine and twelve and happened at three points during the treatment journey over a period of six to twelve months before, during and after management/treatment. Changes were always guided by the pain sufferer and no attempt was made to direct the process into reflecting a 'positive' journey. The lengthy time frame addressed the sense of stasis and paralysis so often accompanying the language and experience of chronic pain.

Sessions usually began by the person with pain talking about their experience. Questions would be posed such as how their pain might be visualised, were there any metaphors they already had for it, could pain be reflected through any particular materials, colours, light—or the absence thereof—or via significant objects they had brought with them. (All participants had been asked to bring in an object which they felt represented something of their experience of pain.) Objects were used to stand in as metaphors for pain, shifting the discussion towards something with personal rather than collective meaning and providing a starting point for the photographic process. Photographs were taken by the artist, using a high-resolution digital camera, in discussion with the person with pain, who often set up the objects within the frame. In subsequent sessions the images would be uploaded onto a computer and reviewed together and discussed. A selection of those deemed successful as photographs and close to the sufferer's experience was later made by artist and patient together. They would either then be modified following the session either by the artist or by the person with pain through printing/

stitching or collaging, or the photograph would be retaken during the next session and refined, as the focus of the image and what an individual wanted it to communicate became more clear. The process brought out the unavoidable relationship between personal narrative and pain experience.

Although predominantly it was objects which were used as metaphors for pain, the photographs produced can also be seen as 'portraits of pain'. Very few participants depicted the actual body, although in some cases the face or body was represented in a figurative way, but usually within metaphoric environments. The images re-enforce Elkin's view that *'every picture is a picture of the body'*[56] though in this context it might be closer to say *'every picture is a picture of the self'*. The process was negotiated differently with each person who participated, and would have been more successful at times than others in re-presenting the illness experience of another 'accurately'.

A selection of the images produced were integrated with images from the earlier *perceptions of pain* project and used to form a pack of pain cards designed as a communication tool for pain clinics. The impact of piloting these cards in the pain clinics of ten experts from a range of specialities is still being analysed, but initial results suggested that changes occur. The images appear to elicit description of the emotional impact and components of pain as well as impacting on non-verbal communication. For example, what is also becoming apparent from observing the consultations is that the space between clinician and patient becomes far more active with greater non-verbal interaction and a more conversational rather than interrogative style of verbal communication. One question is whether this can influence a more negotiated relationship during the rest of the consultation. This is something we are currently exploring in more depth. (For further discussion of their impact on pain consultations please see notes.[57,58,59])

Results of the Co-creative Process

What became interesting was the way that the co-creative process itself generated a different type of language and vocabulary around pain. For example, one patient described how she saw her pain *'as red and black … all distorted and kind of chaotic, and hopeless, an all-consuming kind of thing. It would definitely be something that's fragmented, damaged, torn, destroyed looking … I feel my whole personality, who I am and what I want to do, is destroyed… demolition in progress'* (Fig. 10.1). Another recounted, '*the wires touch each other like this when the pain is most severe*' (Fig. 10.2), another the isolation of when her family were able to go to the gym but she couldn't: '*I can't do anything at the gym, I can't eat healthy fruit. It's like being behind glass or Perspex; a barrier really. When it's not under control I can't do the simplest things. It's this contact with other people. That's the barrier*'. The image-making process as well as the images themselves appeared to shift conversation away from crystallised 'stories' or histories and more towards specific details that individuals wanted or needed to communicate about their pain.

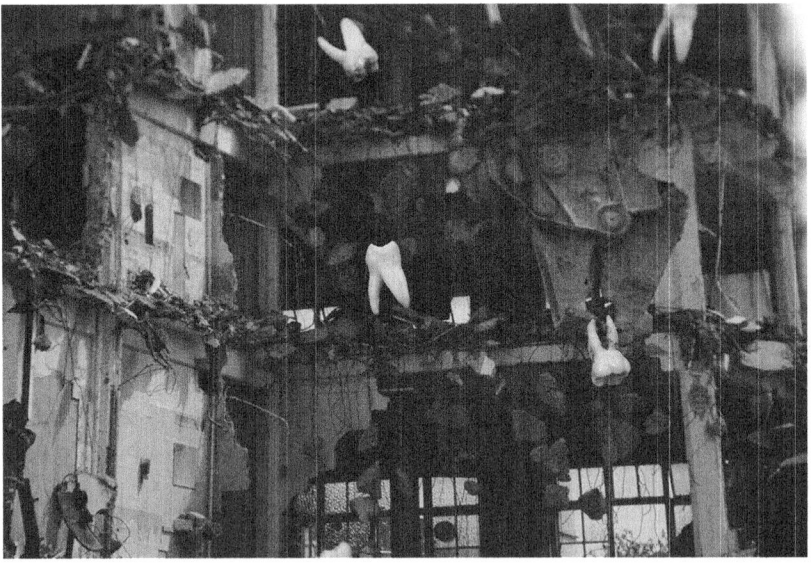

Fig. 10.1 Image of pain co-created by Deborah Padfield with Liz Aldous from the series *face2face*, 2008–2013 © Deborah Padfield

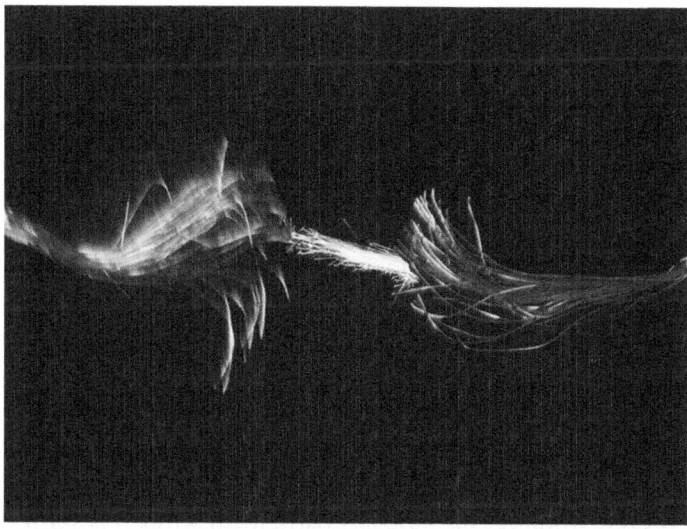

Fig. 10.2 Image of pain co-created by Deborah Padfield with Chandrakant Khoda from the series *face2face*, 2008–2013 © Deborah Padfield

Discussion of the Photograph

Agency, Ambiguity and Specificities of the Photographic Medium

In a paper discussing ways in which photographs can elicit narrative following a study giving cameras to hospital in-patients, social psychologist Alan Radley noted that '*the photographs gained their meaning from the act that produced them; they were not meaningful only in the sense of their pictured content*'.[60] Photography can be seen as not just a medium but as a process, '*a way of making known and shaping experience*'.[61] The fact that pain sufferers were involved in producing the photographs in *face2face* is perhaps important not only to them but to future patients reviewing them in the clinic.

Photographs do not just allow us to recollect personal experience; they also create it. According to photographic theorist John Tagg, the production of images 'animates' rather than 'discovers' meaning.[62,63] It is therefore vital that pain sufferers play an active role in both the creation and the interpretation of images representing their experience. Meaning is being both constructed and revealed during the co-creation process and during review in the clinic. Having control over how their pain and illness is visually represented is essential for any sense of autonomy and wholeness and any sense of responsibility in the recovery process. Control of the lens confers power over how an illness is seen and understood by others, as Jo Spence demonstrated so powerfully with her own illness.[26] By the time pain patients have arrived at a specialist centre, they will almost inevitably have been on the passive receiving end of countless medical imaging processes. Participating in the co-creation of photographic images returns agency, and it is suggested that the process can only be beneficial when sufferers have considerable agency within it. Of her images post-surgery, one *face2face* participant wrote '*I've started drawing where I would like to be after the surgery. I found just what I was looking for, a transparent ball, that I want to put all the photographs and drawings and pins connected with my facial pain inside and have a photograph taken of me kicking it into the distance or throwing it into the air. They are still there, but they are contained within the ball and I can throw it far away. I will have control over it. They will be trapped within the glass and I will be outside of it, instead of behind it*' (Fig. 10.3).

Another reason that photographic images might help negotiate a more 'democratised' interaction in the clinic between patient and clinician might be due to their ambiguity. It is easier to recognise that we all ascribe different interpretations to photographs than to words, even though in the case of the latter it may still be true.[64] Photographs force us to recognise the chasm between our different perspectives and the limits of language available to us to cross this space. As a result we are forced to mediate the image via language and vice versa, to unravel enough meaning to arrive at a shared understanding. Photographs of pain used within medical consultations can help equalise the physical, linguistic and metaphorical space of the consulting room, provoking the co-creation of new ways of 'knowing' illness and pain. Patients used the images to describe pain experience in their own words and its significance for them, for example the image of a broken chain (Fig. 10.4), which had been

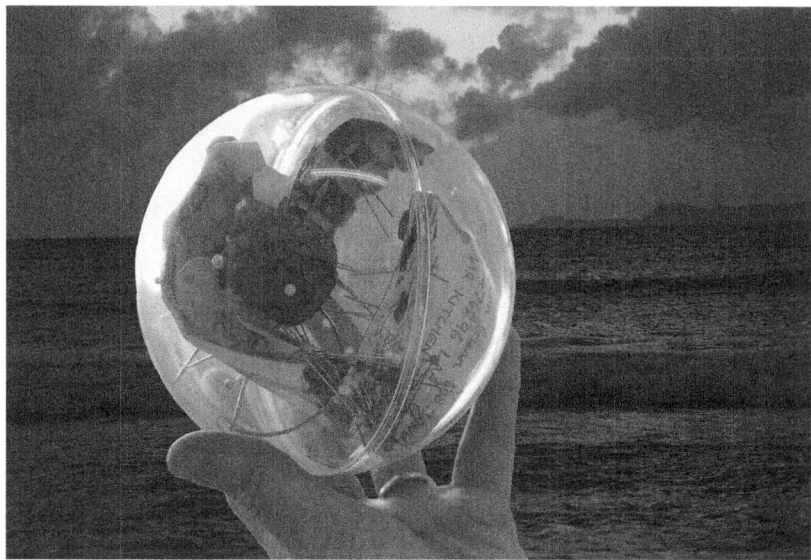

Fig. 10.3 Image of pain co-created by Deborah Padfield with Alison Glenn from the series *face2face*, 2008–2013 © Deborah Padfield

co-created with someone with back pain in the clinic elicited discussion of the gap experienced in family relations: '*and this one it's like a gap, … sometimes I feel a gap between my family … they say they haven't got no time … Christmas as well not all of them is going to come*' (PK3). The same image elicited a different interpretation in another consultation '*it seems that I've got a lot of links that don't connect*' (PC3). One patient used graphic language to describe the quality and impact of pain in response to the photographs '*as if something is being gouged in the ear and twisting round and round, so I picked them for that reason. This one is when it's at its most severest, like knife pains … That's when it gets to the point, I can't take no more*' (PA4), and another frequent refrain '*my GP doesn't listen to me anymore*' (PB3).

The materiality of the photograph as well as its ability to document in some way facilitates empathy and validates the experience of another. Handling the photographs backwards and forwards confers an agency on the images in a Gellian sense—effecting and building social relations.[65] In the following passage the image becomes a shared reference point:

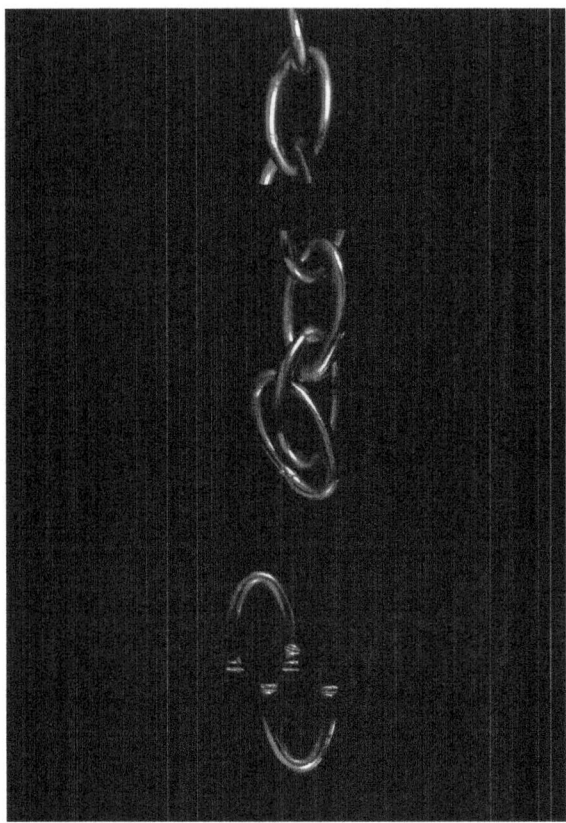

Fig. 10.4 Image of pain co-created by Deborah Padfield with John Pates from the series *perceptions of pain*, 2001–2006 © Deborah Padfield Reproduced by kind permission of Dewi Lewis Publishing

<CH4> *What about this, card number five?*
<PH4> *That would bring tears and weeping from the eye and that.*
<CH4> *Yes, so the electric shock like*
<PH4> *Yes.*
<CH4> *The sparks flying off is, ah, giving me… or telling me a bit about what the pain feels like. Is that what you're getting at?*
<PH4> *That's it, yes.*
<CH4> *Okay. What this about?*
<PH4> *That's with the eye, you know, when it'll hit the eye. I just have to hold my eye. And then this will start weeping and that. The eye will turn red.*

\<CH4\>*Yes.*
\<other UH4\>*Didn't you think when you were embarrassed as well, that, kind of…*
\<PH4\>*Yes, it could be we're sitting having a conversation with you and all of a sudden it would start, just no warning.*
\<CH4\>*Yes. It's quite interesting you mentioned about embarrassment. Tell me a bit more about that.*

In analysing the photographs produced during *Perceptions of Pain*, Cole and Carlin argued images were able to '*span the seemingly unbridgeable gap between the one who suffers pain and the one who hears about pain*'[66] labelling them as '*metaphorical self-portraits*'. The corporeality of the images, the way that the images as photographic objects hold feelings and memories of the body, creates, holds and elicits memory from both patient and clinician. Additionally, the polysemy of photographs allows for a multiplicity of readings revealing what the sufferer/viewer needs to focus on at that moment. We can employ the polysemy of photographs to help us understand experience alien to us, to tolerate complexity and ambiguity, and the pain of not knowing, of not having an answer. Pither[67] argues that clinicians need to help patients as well as themselves to tolerate ambiguity, unknowing and uncertainty. The image-making and image-reviewing processes can allow difficult aspects of experience to enter the discussion which might not easily make their way into a medical space encouraging a toleration of uncertainty.

Face2face: Portraits of Pain: Pain and Identity

The *face2face* images can also be seen as 'portraits of pain'. In a sense, they are the opposite of Mark Gilbert's portraits, which show the visible differences in the faces of patients following maxillofacial surgery.[68] Conversely, the *face2face* photographs focus on and make visible the invisible changes in identity following pain. Very few patients chose to depict the body, though some did (Fig. 10.5). In some ways, the portraits produced are a fusion of objectivities as much as of subjectivities—the distance the photograph provided[69] was used to 'observe', 'witness' and 'unpick' pain experience, rather than present it as fixed and stable. Carlin and Cole

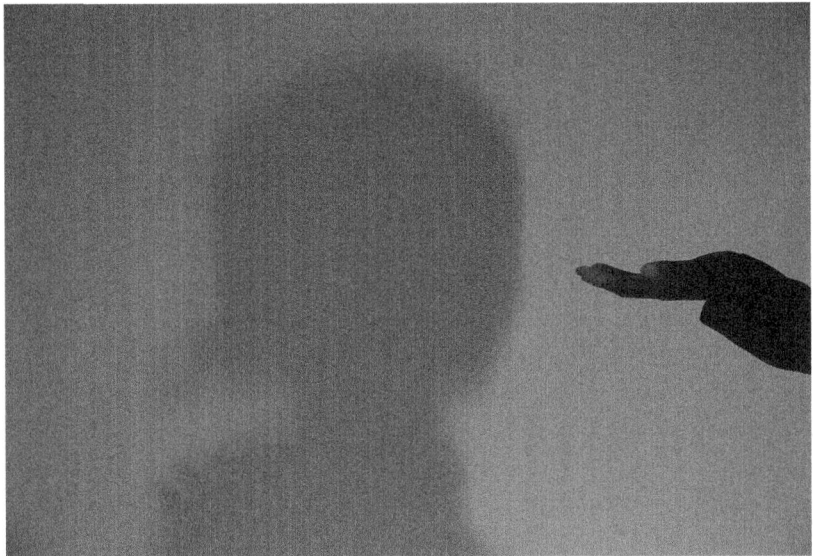

Fig. 10.5 Image of pain co-created by Deborah Padfield with Yante from the series *face2face*, 2008–2013 © Deborah Padfield

support this argument: '*Padfield makes the case for objectifying pain by means of artistic representation so that sufferers can disassociate the pain from their being*'.[70] Photographic portraits and the identities constructed within them are able to remain 'unstable', eliciting different narratives that allow for the possibility of uncertainty and the not yet known—an essential part of being human and perhaps of the chronic pain experience.

This elasticity of identity is further extended through the process of creating multiple portraits over time. Working with people at different points in their pain journey allowed multiple and changing perceptions of pain and identity to emerge. Aspects of experience, which perhaps neither patient nor artist knew were there, could be revealed over time. Could such a reciprocal relationship have implications for the clinician's role in the uncovering of significant narrative *with* and not *for* patients in the context of chronic pain? Directed by the person in pain, the camera allowed significant moments of narrative to be revealed. Kozloff, speaking of Nan Goldin's work, describes a fluidity of 'raw contact'[71] between photographer and subject. The co-creation process at best is an example of raw exchange, capturing through the medium of photography that which is not normally seen; that which is within the power of the subject to choose to reveal or conceal. Jane Fletcher describes the photographic encounter as:

> *two or more people in some sort of dialogue—be it a collaboration or a battle of wills. Two or more people co-operating with or resisting one another.*[72]

It is in a spirit of dialogue that these images are best used in the clinic. In other words, a key contribution of the photograph to the clinic is in the space it creates for negotiation—for unravelling meaning together.

Reflections on the Image in Medicine

In her paper in *Medical Humanities* on how the diagnostic image confronts the lived body in the consulting room, Stahl describes how *'the medical image, presented to the patient by the physician, participates in medicine's cold culture of abstraction, objectification and mandated normativity'*.[73]

From observing the use of the *face2face* images within pain consultations,[9,10,64] it is apparent that conversely photographs of pain co-created with pain sufferers <u>integrate</u> the patient's body into the image, allowing their lived experience to become visible and present in the consulting room, addressing the objectification of which Stahl speaks. The subjective experience of pain can then become shareable within a medical framework as it becomes real and visible to the clinician, currently trained to rely on 'evidence' rather than narrative. Stahl asserts that the medical image *'far from a piece of objective data, testifies to the interplay of particular beliefs, practices and doctrines contemporary medicine holds dear'*, concluding that *'to best treat her patient, the physician must appreciate the influence of these images and appropriately place them within the context of the patient's lived experience*'.[74] In *face2face*, the images were co-created with patients, their selection in clinic made by sufferers, and it is sufferers who influence their interpretation. Thus, instead of testifying to the beliefs of clinicians, they testify to the beliefs of patients.

There is a potency at the intersection of pain, language and image where new language can be born from patients' own social and linguistic worlds, which would not only allow patients but also clinicians to tolerate the uncertain, irrational nature of pain experience and move forward together in discussing its management in the context of that individual patient's life.

Conclusion

Photographic images can give tangible form to confusing sensations, providing a shared aesthetic space within which to negotiate, both with the 'other' and with one's attachment to previously held perceptions. It is the collaborative search for meaning they stimulate within the consulting room which potentially validates the pain cards as a communication tool.

Bleakley argues '*Medicine must democratise ... improved communication lowers patient risk in reducing medical error. The arts ... provide the media through which such democratisation can be learned*'.[75]

Face2face is the first in-depth project to study the impact of using photographs of pain as an intervention in clinician-patient dialogue across a multi-disciplinary team of experts in an NHS hospital using video recordings which can be compared with self-reporting evaluation forms. From the results beginning to emerge, the images appear to generate new language enriching pain descriptions and facilitating discussion of emotional aspects of pain significant to its intensity and prolongation for that individual. They could also play a role in teaching healthcare professionals to raise awareness of chronic pain and its attendant suffering. We suggest these early findings warrant further interdisciplinary analysis/investigation to assess and validate the images as a new communication tool for improving doctor-patient dialogue across the NHS and argue that photographic images and image-making processes should be considered valuable tools for democratising medical pain encounters.

Notes

1. Hjermstad, M. J., P. M. Fayers, D. F. Haugen, et al. "Studies Comparing Numerical Rating Scales, Verbal Rating Scales, and Visual Analogue Scales for Assessment of Pain Intensity in Adults: A Systematic Literature Review". *Journal of Pain and Symptom Management* 41 (2011): 1073–1093.
2. Morse, J. M. "Using Qualitative Methods to Access the Pain Experience". *British Journal of Pain* 9 (2015): 26–31.
3. Deignan, A, J. Littlemore, and E. Semino, eds. *Figurative Language, Genre and Register* (Cambridge: Cambridge University Press, 2013), 267–304.
4. Scarry, E. *The Body in Pain: The Making and Unmaking of the World* (Oxford: Oxford University Press, 1985).
5. Charon, R. "A Narrative Medicine for Pain". In *Narrative Pain and Suffering: Progress in Pain Research and Management*, edited by D. Carr, J. Loeser, and D. Morris, vol. 34 (Seattle: IASP Press, 2005).
6. Biro, D. *The Language of Pain. Finding Words, Compassion and Relief* (New York: WW Norton & Co, 2010).
7. Bourke, J. *Pain and the Politics of Sympathy, Historical Reflections, 1760s to 1960s* (Utrecht: Universiteit Utrecht, 2011), 10. *Back to Context.*
8. Padfield, D. "Mask: Mirror: Membrane". *Pain News* 10, no. 2 (2012): 104–109.
9. Padfield, D. Unpublished PhD dissertation, University College London, 2013.
10. Padfield, D., J. M. Zakrzewska, and A. C. de C. Williams. "Do Photographic Images of Pain Improve Communication During Pain Consultations?" *Pain Research & Management* 20, no. 3 (2015): 123–128.
11. Padfield, D. *Perceptions of Pain.* 1st ed. (Stockport: Dewi Lewis Publishing, 2003).
12. Padfield, D, F. Janmohamed, and J. M. Zakrzewska, et al. "A Slippery Surface, Can Photographic Images of Pain Improve Communication in Pain Consultations?" *International Journal of Surgery* 8, no. 2 (2010): 144–150.
13. Bleakley, A. Association of Medical Humanities Conference Programme, 2015: 3.
14. Biro, D. "Psychological Pain: Metaphor or Reality?" In *Pain and Emotion in Modern History*, edited by R. Boddice (Basingstoke: Palgrave Macmillan, 2014), 53–65.

15. Biro (6): 104. Craig and Williams have also recently proposed expanding the IASP definition of pain to include a distressing experience associated with actual or potential tissue damage with sensory, emotional, cognitive and social components (A. C. de. C. Williams and K. D. Craig. *Updating the Definition of Pain: Pain* 157 (2016): 2420–2423.
16. Bourke, J. *The Story of Pain: From Prayer to Painkillers* (Oxford: Oxford University Press, 2014).
17. Good, B. J. *Medicine, Rationality, and Experience: An Anthropological Perspective* (Cambridge: Cambridge University Press, 1994).
18. Boddice, R., ed. *Pain and Emotion in Modern History* (Basingstoke: Palgrave Macmillan, 2014).
19. Kleinman, A. *The Illness Narratives, Suffering, Healing & the Human Condition* (USA: Basic Books, 1988).
20. Kleinman, A. "Catastrophe and Caregiving: The Failure of Medicine as an Art". *Lancet* 371 (2008): 22–23.
21. Kleinman, A. "Care: In Search of a Health Agenda". *Lancet* 386 (2015): 240–241.
22. Green, C. R. "Being Present: The Role of Narrative Medicine in Reducing the Unequal Burden of Pain". *Pain* 152 (2011): 965–966.
23. Charon (5): 29.
24. Charon (5): 30.
25. Harrison, B. "Seeing Health and Illness Worlds—Using Visual Methodologies in a Sociology of Health and Illness: A Methodological Review". *Sociology of Health & Illness* 24, no. 6 (2002): 856.
26. Spence, J. *Putting Myself in the Picture* (London: Camden Press, 1986).
27. Martin, R., and J. Spence. "New Portraits for Old: The Use of Camera in Therapy". In *Looking on: Images of Femininity in the Visual Arts and Media*, edited by R. Betterton (London: Pandora, 1987), 267–279.
28. Dennett, T., "Jo Spence's Auto-therapeutic Survival Strategies". In Bell, S., and A. Radley, eds. "Representations of Illness and Disease". *Health* 15, no. 3 (2011): 223–239.
29. Radley, A., and D. Taylor. "Images of Recovery: A Photoelicitation Study on the Hospital Ward". *Qualitative Health Research* 13 (2003): 77–99.
30. Radley, A., D. Hodgetts, and A. Cullen. "Visualising Homelessness: A Study of Photography and Estrangement". *Journal of Community and Applied Social Psychology* 15 (2005): 273–295.
31. Radley, A. *Works of Illness: Narrative, Picturing and the Social Response to Serious Disease* (Ashby–de-la-Zouch, UK: InkerMen Press, 2009).

32. Radley, A. "What People Do with Pictures". *Visual Studies* 25, no. 3 (2010): 268–279.
33. Henriksen, N., T. Tjornhoj-Thomsen, H. Ploug Hansen. "Illness, Everyday Life and Narrative Montage: The Visual Aesthetics of Cancer in Sara Bro's Diary". In Bell, S., and A. Radley, eds. "Representations of Illness and Disease". *Health* 15, no. 3 (2011): 277–297.
34. Willenfelt, J. "Documenting Bodies: Pain Surfaces". In *Pain and Emotion in Modern History*, edited by R. Boddice (Basingstoke; New York: Palgrave Macmillan, 2014), 260–276 (or do I use Boddice (18) here?).
35. Collen, M. "Life of Pain, Life of Pleasure: Pain from the Patients' Perspective – The Evolution of the PAIN Exhibit". *Journal of Pain & Palliative Care Pharmacotherapy* 19, no. 4 (2005): 45–52.
36. Collen, M. PAIN. http://painexhibit.org/ accessed 5th August 2014.
37. Main, S. "Picturing Pain: Using Creative Methods to Communicate the Experience of Chronic Pain". *Pain News* no. 1 (2012): 32–35. http://www.britishpainsociety.org/bps_nl_vol12_issue1.pdf
38. Gonzalez-Polledo, E., and J. Tarr. "The Thing About Pain: The Remaking of Illness Narratives in Chronic Pain Expression on Social Media". *Newmedia & Society* (2014): 1–18.
39. Davis, F. D. "The Problem of Pain". In *Maldynia, Multidisciplinary Perspectives on the Illness of Chronic Pain*, edited by J. Giordano (New York: Taylor & Francis, 2011), 243–255.
40. Wilkinson, M., and D. Robinson. "Migraine Art". *Cephalalgia* 5, no. 3 (1985): 151–157.
41. Broadbent, E., K. Niederhoffer, and T. Hague, et al. "Headache Sufferers' Drawings Reflect Distress, Disability and Illness Perceptions". *Journal of Psychosomatic Research* 66 (2009): 465–470.
42. Maclean, S. "Exploring the Use of Drawings for Patients Communicating Chronic Pain to Healthcare Professionals". *Pain News* Winter (2009): 34–37. http://www.britishpainsociety.org/bps_nl_winter_2009.pdf
43. Geller, B. "The PainT project". *Pain News* Winter (2011): 42–43. http://www.britishpainsociety.org/bps_nl_winter_2011.pdf
44. McMahon, E., L. Wilson-Pauwels, J. Henry, et al. "The Iconic Pain Assessment Tool: Facilitating the Translation of Pain Sensations and Improving Patient-Physician Dialogue". *Journal of Bio-Communication* 34, no. 2 (2008): E20–E24.
45. Lalloo, C., and J. L. Henry. "Evaluation of the Iconic Pain Assessment Tool by a Heterogeneous Group of People in Pain". *Pain Research and Management* 16, no. 1 (2011): 13–18.

46. Stones, C. "Positively Picturing Pain? Using Patient-Generated Pictures to Establish Affective Visual Design Qualities". *International Journal of Design* 7, no. 1 (2013): 85–97.
47. Closs, S. J., P. Knapp, S. Morely, et al. "Can Pictorial Images Communicate the Quality of Pain Successfully?" *British Journal of Pain* (2015): 1–8.
48. Dannequin, L. *Hardy Animal*. AMH Conference 2015.
49. Eisenberger, N. I., M. D. Lieberman, and K. D. Williams. "Does Rejection Hurt? An FMRI Study of Social Exclusion". *Science* 302, no. 5643 (2003): 290–292.
50. Tracey, I. "Objectifying Pain Through Brain Imaging". In *Narrative Pain and Suffering: Progress in Pain Research and Management*, edited by D. Carr, J. Loeser, and D. Morris, vol. 34 (Seattle, USA: IASP Press, 2005), 137.
51. Carr, D., J. Loeser, and D. Morris, eds. *Narrative Pain and Suffering: Progress in Pain Research and Management*. Vol. 34 (Seattle, USA: IASP Press, 2015).
52. Tracey, I., and P. Mantyh. "The Cerebral Signature for Pain Perception and Its Modulation". *Neuron* 55(Aug. 2, 2007): 377–391.
53. Wiech, K., and I. Tracey. "The Influence of Negative Emotions on Pain: Behavioral Effects and Neural Mechanisms". *NeuroImage* 47 (2009): 987–994.
54. McMahon, S. B., and M. Koltzenburg. *Textbook of Pain*. 5th ed. (London: Elsevier, 2006).
55. Jones, D. "Portraits of Pain". *Lancet* 378, no. 9789 (July 30, 2011): 391.
56. Elkins, J. *Pictures of the Body: Pain and Metamorphosis* (Stanford: Stanford University Press,1999): 1.
57. Padfield, D., and J. M. Zakrzewska. "Encountering Pain". *Lancet* 2017: 389 (in press).
58. Semino, E., J. M. Zakrzewska, and A. Williams. "Images and the Dynamic of Pain Consultations". *Lancet* 389 (2017): 1186–1187.
59. Padfield, D., T. Chadwick, and H. Omand. "The Body as Image: Image as Body" 2017: 389 (in press).
60. Radley (44): 270.
61. Radley (44): 270.
62. Tagg, J. "Power and Photography: Part One, A Means of Surveillance: The Photograph as Evidence in Law". *Screen Education* 36 (autumn 1980): 17–55.
63. Tagg, J. *The Disciplinary Frame: Photographic Truths and the Capture of Meaning* (Minneapolis: University of Minnesota Press, 2009), 1.

64. Padfield, D. "Representing the 'Pain of Others'". In Bell, S., and A. Radley, eds. "Another Way of Knowing; Art, Disease and Illness". *Health* 15, no. 3 (2011): 241–258.
65. Gell, A. *Art and Agency, An Anthropological Theory* (New York; Oxford: Clarendon Press, 1998).
66. Carlin, N., and T. Cole. "Maldynia as Muse: A Recent Experiment in the Visual Arts and Medical Humanities. In *Maldynia, Multidisciplinary Perspectives on the Illness of Chronic Pain*, ed. J. Giordano (New York: Taylor & Francis, 2011), 105. 67.
67. Pither, C. "Pain Clinic is Not a Place for Diagnosis". *Pain News* (Winter 2011): 21.
68. Gilbert, M. *Saving Faces*. Exhibition of portraits by Mark Gilbert. National Portrait Gallery, London, 2002.
69. Sontag, S. *On Photography* (London: Penguin, 1978).
70. Carlin & Cole (20): 105.
71. Kosloff, M. "Real Faces". In *Lone Visions, Crowded Frames: Essays on Photography* (Albuquerque: University of New Mexico Press, 1994), 76–78.
72. Fletcher, J. "Sweet Liberties: Narratives of Resistance and Desire". In *Masquerade: Women's Contemporary Portrait Photography*, edited by K. Newton and C. Rolph (Cardiff: Ffotogallery Publishing, 2003), 51.
73. Stahl, D. "Living into the Imagined Body: How the Diagnostic Image Confronts the Lived Body". *Medical Humanities* 39 (2013): 53–58.
74. Stahl (84): 53–54.
75. Bleakley (13): 11.

Acknowledgments This work was completed as part of Deborah Padfield's PhD thesis under the primary supervision of Prof Sharon Morris, Slade Deputy Director, Slade School of Fine Art. Her PhD was funded by the Arts and Humanities Research Council, UK. We are grateful to all the patients and clinicians who participated in the study and to Prof Alan Radley and Dr Deborah Kirklin for their valuable comments on earlier drafts.

Competing Interests Neither of the authors has any conflict of interest to disclose.

Funding Arts & Humanities Research Council (AHRC) and Arts Council England (ACE). Deborah Padfield was supported by the AHRC and by a Centre for Humanities Interdisciplinary Research Fellowship (CHIRP) from University College London (UCL), and Joanna Zakrzewska was supported by the National Institute for Health Research University College London Hospitals (UCLH) Biomedical Research Centre while carrying out this research.

The multidisciplinary analyses were supported by the Friends UCH and by Grand Challenges, UCL.

Deborah Padfield is a visual artist specialising in lens-based media. She is currently a Teaching Fellow and Honorary Research Associate at the Slade School of Fine Art, UCL. In 2001, her collaboration with Dr Charles Pither at St Thomas' Hospital led to a touring exhibition and a book, *Perceptions of Pain*. Her recent collaboration with Professor Joanna Zakrzewska and facial pain clinicians and patients from UCLH led to several exhibitions, symposia, their current project *Pain: speaking the threshold* and several publications including a series of essays in the *Lancet*. She is the recipient of a number of awards including Sciart Research Award, UCL Arts in Health Award, the UCL Provost's Award for Public Engagement 2012, British Pain Society Artist of the Year 2012 and a UCL Public Engagement Beacon Bursary 2015.

Joanna M. Zakrzewska obtained dental (Kings College, London) and medical (Cambridge) degrees and specialist training in oral medicine, going on to specialise in orofacial pain and become a fellow of the Faculty of Pain Medicine. As Professor of Pain Medicine she led a multidisciplinary facial pain unit at UCLH NHS Foundation Trust, London for seven years, where she now holds a part-time appointment. She is now setting up a national centre for trigeminal neuralgia. Joanna is working with Deborah Padfield, a visual artist, to determine how photography could enable improved communication about pain. She has written four books, 24 chapters and over 100 papers. She lectures extensively, both nationally and internationally.

11

Painscapes and Method

Jen Tarr

Pain, Language and Method

In this volume, we have developed the concept of painscapes to refer to multiple ways of seeing and navigating pain. For Appadurai, the suffix '-scape' indicates 'first of all that these are not objectively given relations which look the same from every angle of vision, but rather that they are deeply perspectval constructs, inflected very much by the historical, linguistic and political situatedness of different sorts of actors'.[1] Painscapes are 'imagined worlds', worlds in which different aspects of pain—as personal, societal, private, public—are foregrounded. While the actors at work in chronic pain may be different than those in Appadurai's '-scapes', they are equally situated, equally perspectval. What we see about chronic pain depends on the lens through which we view the painscape, but also upon the angle, the direction and the distance from which we are viewing. In what follows, I will argue for the value—indeed the necessity—of

J. Tarr (✉)
London School of Economics and Political Science, London, UK

© The Author(s) 2018
EJ Gonzalez-Polledo, J. Tarr (eds.), *Painscapes*,
https://doi.org/10.1057/978-1-349-95272-4_11

interdisciplinarity in relation to pain. I begin with the challenge so frequently discussed in work on pain communication, of pain's fraught relationship to language, arguing that it is method rather than language that pain resists, at least insofar as this refers to a fixed, linear and reproducible way of working. I suggest that by taking method back to its etymological roots as a 'way of travelling', we can more successfully navigate the diverse fields—the painscapes—with which pain presents us.

Probably the most quoted lines from Elaine Scarry's book *The Body in Pain* are those where she speaks about language, remarking that

> for the person in pain so incontestably and unnegotiably present is it that 'having pain' may come to be thought of as the most vibrant example of what it is to 'have certainty', while for the other person it is so elusive that 'hearing about pain' may exist as the primary model of what it is 'to have doubt' ...Whatever pain achieves, it achieves in part through its unsharability, and it ensures this unsharability through its resistance to language.[2]

She goes on to add that 'Physical pain does not simply resist language but actively destroys it, bringing about an immediate reversion to a state anterior to language, to the sounds and cries a human being makes before language is learned'.[3]

Scarry's statement has been influential because it seems intuitively correct: pain is difficult to speak about, and it can feel impossible to know anything about the pain that another person is experiencing. Yet a great deal of scholarly work has emerged from a variety of fields, from literature[4] to history[5] to sociology,[6] suggesting that expression in language is important, indeed central, to the experience of pain. Wittgenstein's 'pain and private language' argument suggests that in order to be expressed or communicated, pain requires language and social interaction. As Bourke summarises: 'the naming of a "pain-event" can never be wholly private. Although pain is generally regarded as a subjective phenomenon—it possesses a "mine-ness"—naming occurs in public realms[7]'. Bourke highlights the role of metaphor in shaping how pain is conceptualised, and how the metaphors used to communicate pain have shifted over time and across cultures. Changes in the metaphorical language of pain have occurred due to changing conceptions of bodily physiology, developments in the external environment such as shifts towards mechanisation and industrialisation and broader ideological shifts. The language of pain is far from universal: Bourke points out, for instance, that the McGill Pain Questionnaire's English-language associations between pain and punishment were incomprehensible to Finnish speakers when researchers attempted to translate it.[8]

Beyond everyday linguistic expressions, science and medicine have also had a difficult time pinning down pain. While we commonly understand pain to correlate with injury or damage to a part of the body, there are many cases of pain in the absence of injury; injury in the absence of pain; and cases where the location of pain does not correlate with the location of injury, to name but a few issues. 'If the study of pain in people is to have a scientific foundation, it is essential to measure it. If we want to know how effective a new drug is, we need numbers to say that the pain decreased by some amount', argue foundational pain researchers Melzack and Wall.[9] They point to the McGill Pain Questionnaire[10,11] as a tool for doing this because it is an advance on previous versions of pain measurement that allow only for variations in intensity. They note that 'to describe pain solely in terms of intensity is like specifying the visual world only in terms of light flux without regard to pattern, colour, texture, and the many other dimensions of visual experience'.[12] For Melzack and Wall, the attempt to make a more nuanced language of pain available is a key step in making pain more scientifically accessible. The MPQ has been designed to provide reliable, repeatable measures and descriptions of pain, to augment intensity-based scales such as the Numerical Rating Scale, Visual Analogue Scale, Colour Analogue scale or the 'Faces' scale[13] often used with children in which a series of progressively unhappy faces are used to depict the severity of the pain.

Crawford has argued that rather than resisting language, 'the perception, performance, meaning, and effects of pain are constituted in and through shared discourses'.[14] To demonstrate this she traces the history of how phantom limb sensations were presented in medical literature. In the 1950s and earlier, the tingling associated with them was often described as pleasurable or pleasant, whereas from the 1970s onward the associated sensation is far more frequently described as pain. Crawford points to the role of the McGill Pain Questionnaire in shaping pain's linguistic expression, and shows that the language associated with phantom limb sensations after the widespread adoption of the MPQ in 1975 is consonant with that instrument. She challenges Melzack's claim to have established a relatively universal language of pain descriptors whose provision patients are relieved to be offered:

> Aside from the unanswered methodological question of how a physician might know the very words that he or she does not have access to, what is of significance here is that these descriptors are constructed as 'acceptable' and 'sound' based on the administrator's sense of the patient's relief. It is not that one should warily accept that patients are genuinely relieved to establish a shared understanding of their pain experience, but rather that the administrator qua instrument is tapping into something authentic, something 'out there', something static, when in fact it is more accurate to say that the MPQ functions to construct the qualitative dimensions of a language of pain.[15]

Standardised pain measurement tools have been critiqued widely, even as they continue to have prevalence. De Souza and Frank[16] discovered that patients' own spontaneous pain descriptors differed from those on the MPQ, with words like 'shouting' or 'red' indicating dimensions not considered by Melzack. Williams, Davies and Chadury[17] found that patients often make sense of pain scales in idiosyncratic ways, for instance by thinking through functionality or mobility when they assess whether their pain is a '1' or a '10' and weighing, for example, whether one part of the body is more painful than another and if so, which pain they should report on. Smith[18] found that notes from respondents in the margins of pain questionnaires served many of the same functions, calling forth an 'imagined researcher' who would be able to help interpret the vagaries of their pain experience and from there determine whether they had answered the questions in the desired way. Litcher-Kelly and colleagues found that clinical trials and randomised controlled trials of pain treatments tended to use unidimensional measures of pain, most frequently the Visual Analogue Scale.[19] Moreover, there was little consistency in the tools used, with 28 different pain outcome tools being used across 50 studies. Despite pain's multidimensional nature, then, many potential treatments are still not being evaluated in terms of their impact across pain's 'sensory, affective, behavioural, social and attitudinal factors', but only in terms of potential reduction of intensity, a measure which is at best partial and at worst woefully inadequate.

In an illustrative passage in her book on living with chronic pain, Lou Heshusius describes her thought processes on being given a Numerical Rating Scale by her clinician:

> Here we go again. What to mark. Last time I think I said my pain was a 6. But I don't exactly remember how bad the pain was when I circled a 6. Or, I think: I feel only light pain right now. Perhaps I feel a 3. But five minutes from now it may be a 2 or a 4. Becoming impatient with the scale and my inability to get it 'right'—because getting it right is impossible—I just circle a 3. Done. I give the whole thing back to the secretary.[20]

As these examples suggest, pain's challenges go beyond merely the problem of linguistic representation and resistance: pain perpetually resists attempts to standardise and measure it in any consistent, coherent way. While these tools have been validated and shown to produce relatively stable results, they are often unsatisfactory for patients and fail to capture the feeling of living with pain and the myriad ways it affects one's life. In short, what pain resists is not simply language, but also method. The search for method as a replicable, repeatable path is one performed throughout medicine as well as in much social science. These paths have value, but they also limit our findings and what it becomes possible to say about pain: to that which can be documented on a questionnaire, quantified on a Numerical Rating Scale or Visual Analogue Scale,[21] marked on a pain drawing during clinical assessment,[22] or expressed in standardised language.[10,11]

But what is a method? Etymologically, the word derives from the Latin *methodus*: 'a way of teaching or going'. Originally, one of its references was to a path or journey, a way of travelling. This is particularly apt in light of the concept of painscapes we have proposed. Like a landscape, encountered on a journey, method provides a path, a way through the painscape which can be charted, followed by others. In what follows, I will outline several alternative paths I have taken through pain research, attempting to bring visual and other sensory methods to bear on pain's invisibility. While each of these presents an alternative version of pain to that outlined in clinical practice, every method has drawbacks, things it silences or makes invisible in the process of bringing other things to the fore. My argument is not for triangulation in the classical sense, but for multiplicity, and for recognition of the 'messiness'[23] of phenomena like pain. I suggest that by recognising our methods as ways of travelling, we can better acknowledge the range of journeys it is necessary to make in order to understand pain.

Paths Through Researching Pain Experience

I first began researching pain in the context of a project on dancers' experiences of pain and injury. Our project was set against the context that injury rates amongst professional dancers are very high, with around 80–85 per cent of UK dancers self-reporting injury in any given year.[24,25] Of those injuries, the majority are chronic rather than acute.[26] It is therefore likely that many of them were associated with pain before they crossed the threshold into being defined as injuries. But where is that threshold? What makes a dancer decide that something is an injury rather than merely an ongoing pain or 'niggle', or the 'good pain' they associate with training? Our research used a multi-method approach, drawing on cultural phenomenology to try to make sense of how dancers distinguish between pain and injury, and the consequences this has for their bodies and careers. A total of 205 dancers answered a brief questionnaire and then took part in a qualitative interview, followed by a body mapping process using 3D images of themselves generated in a white light body scanner and manipulated through computer software.

Each of these methods produced different results: reports of pain and injury on questionnaires at the beginning of the interview process contrasted with the images created at the end of the process. The questionnaires indicated that 90 per cent of dancers in the study had been injured at some point in their careers. By the end of the body mapping process that number had increased to 97 per cent. A total of 46 dancers claimed to have had no recent pain and 21 claimed to have never been injured. From the body maps, 34 of the 46 marked recent pain on the maps, while six of the 'uninjured' participants went on to mark injuries. Many of those who said they had only been injured once or twice went on to mark far more than one or two sites of injury. For those who had marked five or six injuries, in some cases fewer injuries were marked on the body map than had been listed on the questionnaire. Overall, however, the trend was towards increased marking of pain and injury on the body maps as compared to the initial questionnaires.

Why did these methods not triangulate? Was it merely a case of desirability bias: did participants, in the course of an interview on pain and injury, reframe some experiences as injury in order to have more to represent or draw? Did they see this as part of 'being a good participant'? It is possible that this happened in a few cases, but far more frequent in the interviews was evidence that they remembered old injuries through talking about them—often major injuries such as broken bones and torn cartilage. In total, the interview transcripts included 32 incidents of dancers remembering injuries through the interviews that they had previously forgotten. The mapping process, which required 'thinking through the body' as they literally scanned, patted and manipulated parts of their bodies in order to remember past pains and injuries, enabled further remembering.

In other cases, dancers redefined ongoing pains as injuries, confronted with evidence that these pains closely resembled their definitions of injury. The process of being asked to articulate what constituted an injury and how it was different from pain caused many to rethink their distinctions in the final act of producing a body map. The process of qualitative interviewing, recalling and discussing their experiences of injury and ongoing, chronic pains made them reconsider where the boundaries were between pain and injury and how their own experiences fit with the definitions they had given. Many held competing or disparate definitions of pain or injury. For instance, some described injury as something that impaired function, but they might also define it as something that stopped them from dancing, or something that was diagnosed as injury by a medical professional, or something acute, that you 'would know right away' when it had happened. A particular pain might indeed impair function, even preventing dancing, but if it had not had a formal diagnosis and/or if it had come on slowly, as many overuse injuries do, the dancer might never have identified it as an injury.

One dancer, for example, defined injury as something acute that was diagnosed as such by a health professional, but also knew intellectually that this this was not an adequate or accurate definition:

> Diana[27]: I'm still a bit, I guess immature about that one. I'm still not completely clear about that. I hope that when I'll be, like I say, I think for me injured is when you're in hospital and the doctor tells you this is broken or this is sprained or you need surgery, like that's an injury. And because I've never, thank God, experienced that then for me I never considered being injured.

She had, however, continued to dance with ongoing, crippling back pain that had a significant effect on her daily life outside of class. By the final mapping process, after a discussion in which she articulated a shifting awareness and a process of coming to be somewhat more careful with her body, she chose to mark the back pain as a past injury.

In sports science, there is evidence that injury recall after more than twelve months is weak when measured by self-reporting on questionnaires.[28] This suggests that alternative methods are needed for gaining a more accurate or adequate picture of experiences of injury, something our body mapping tool may provide. Yet the body scanning and mapping process was by no means a neutral instrument. We became aware early in the process that dancers' self-representation was as much about their perceptions and desired self-presentation as it was about an accurate view of their bodies. This was particularly the case when they marked areas of perceived strength and weakness. Some dancers, especially those with ongoing pain or injuries, marked large portions of their body as weak and very few, if any, as strong. Other dancers marked many areas of strength, including one man who painted his entire body green (the colour that represented strength), marking injuries and pain merely with small dots on the affected joints! As an ageing male dancer who had succeeded in pursuing a career long past when many colleagues had retired, he was proud of his achievements and wanted to emphasise his strength rather than focusing on weakness, pain or injury. In seeing the scan images of themselves, dancers also regularly commented on the shape and size of their bodies as represented by the scanner, and any discrepancies or unevenness between sides. Their responses to the body mapping itself were mainly positive: they called it an amazing tool, said it made them more aware or that they remembered more when they were seeing the scan, that they found it fascinating to see themselves represented in this way or that it showed them what they needed to work on. Two dancers said that they could actually feel the pain whilst they marked it on the image. For others, however, the experience was less positive: they said they already knew their bodies well and didn't notice anything new, or that 'it doesn't feel like my body'. A few described it as 'not nice' or 'creepy' to see their bodies represented so starkly.

The problems became more serious with other dancers, as we have documented elsewhere.[29] The scanner's software was programmed to recognise a particular version of a body: something with two arms and legs, capable of standing upright, responding to audio cues, and with a relatively high contrast between their skin tone and the black backdrop of the scanner. Poorer quality images were produced of anyone who did not meet these criteria. This was particularly problematic in the case of dancers with disabilities, when we had to 'trick' the scanner into believing they had all their limbs or could stand without support. While our research aimed to examine experiences of embodiment, the experience of the body scanner could also be quite disembodying for some participants.

As this project came to an end, I became interested in how images were used in pain mapping more broadly and in what kinds of images might be most useful. Did the three-dimensionality of the images make a difference? Did it matter if the images were of the participants themselves? Would line drawings be as useful and effective? With these questions in mind, and aiming to produce versions of pain mapping that would be more inclusive and accessible than our work with the body scanner, I began a pilot project on pain and visual mapping. Seven participants—people with pain, both dancers and non-dancers, with and without disabilities—participated in group or individual interviews and mapping processes in which they could choose to mark a line drawing, sculpt a version of themselves with plasticine modelling clay, and/or mark pain on a digital image of themselves. What they chose to mark and how they described their experiences was left up to them.

Although this study involved only a few participants, their pain descriptors were enlightening and served to further complicate my understanding of the relation between pain and method. Two participants, non-dancers who experienced osteoarthritis, lacked ways of describing pain. Their maps were relatively sparse, limited to two colours and sensations. One participant's arthritis affected his hands so badly that he was not able to model the clay or use the computer mouse to mark an image of himself. This was an important reminder that even less sophisticated technologies can enable some participants while disabling others. This participant was nonetheless highly aware of the exact location of the pain, and he directed me precisely as to where to mark pain on the digital image. The second participant with osteoarthritis, when asked to think about visual images related to her pain, remarked thoughtfully:

> Elise: I've never thought about it visually. This is problematic. I've never thought about it belonging to a part of my body, it's simply that arthritic pain in my knee, that arthritic pain because it's the same sort of pain but it's in various different parts of my body. So I'm not thinking of my body, I'm thinking of the pain. So that's a kind of entity in and of itself.

This arthritic pain was not the same as previous ongoing pain she had experienced due to a slipped disc. These pains, however, were described by cause rather than sensation, marked as 'slipped disc', 'arthritis' and 'broken bones' on her pain maps. Similarly, the second participant with osteoarthritis also described pain in functional terms related to diagnosis. This was in contrast to the participants who were dancers, whose descriptions were more elaborate and elaborated. For dancers without disabilities, pain was subdivided into types: 'injury pain', 'nerve pain', 'skin pain', 'old pain', 'historic', 'core' or 'edges' of pain and injury, 'mild pain', 'inflexibility pain' and 'pressure pain'. Those with disabilities had descriptors that overlapped and also extended their colleagues' descriptors: several also referred to the cause of the pain ('tension due to spasticity caused by disability'; 'neuro pain', 'internal organ pain'), while others described areas of stiffness and strength. Two participants with cerebral palsy each described some types of pain as 'necessary' or 'manageable'.

How participants interpreted the array of images with which they were provided depended then on their daily use of their bodies and the frequency with which they encountered the limits of pain: what were they asking of themselves? Did pain differ in different contexts? Both able-bodied and disabled dancers, who had ongoing daily involvement with their bodies, indicated far more detailed mental maps of pain gradations and distinctions than the two participants with osteoarthritis, for whom pain had only a few dimensions. Form dictated direction.

For one participant, the process of sculpting herself in plasticine was the one that best evoked her sense of her own embodied experience. The small figure evoked protective feelings; it made her realise what she was doing to herself when she pushed her body to work with pain and injury and made her want to reconsider doing so. She was able to identify with the figure, and it made her want to be more careful with herself as well as with the figure. The figure became imbued with some sense of herself:

> Fiona: [You] can abuse your body, but when you're in charge of it in some sort of detached way, like with the model, you suddenly realise this is my body, like what am I doing? …Which I wouldn't have predicted, but now I kind of look and say you don't want those red splodges [of pain] or something, let's not have those. And so it kind of makes me more aware that it doesn't need to be, you don't need to be in pain if you can get out of it somehow.

To Elise, the participant quoted earlier, however, the model seemed too subjective and too dependent on one's ability to sculpt. For her, filling in the standard blank figure on the pain drawing was the most useful form of pain mapping.

The project therefore underscored the ways that pain and other bodily sensations are interpreted differently depending on context. How would the pain descriptors above fit with standardised forms of measurement such as the McGill Pain Questionnaire? Where within a pain survey would descriptions such as 'necessary' or 'manageable' come in? Like the respondents Smith (2008) described, participants felt compelled to describe and explain what they meant by different sensations, and in some cases to incorporate elaborate and nuanced distinctions between different types of pain: from 'core' and 'edges' of pains and injury, both past and present, to 'areas of strength that allow me to compensate for weak areas' and 'areas of tension due to spasticity caused by disability—but they are manageable'.

The most recent research project, *Communicating Chronic Pain: Interdisciplinary Strategies for Non-Textual Data*, took up the problem of pain and method from a different angle: what could sensory and arts-based approaches offer to the study of chronic pain communication? How might they enable chronic pain to be communicated, or indeed conceived, differently?

The research examined non-textual expressions of chronic pain on social media, looking at Flickr and Tumblr.[30,31] It also aimed to create new non-textual forms of pain expression by undertaking workshops with artists, people with pain, and clinicians. The workshops explored drawing, sculpting, digital photography, sound and physical theatre, with a pair of workshop leaders skilled in the relevant methods leading groups of people with pain, a handful of interested clinicians, and the research team through a series of activities and exercises. Each workshop began with a round of introductions, followed by some initial explorations of the materials under discussion. This might include a round of taking photographs, trying out different kinds of sounds, or theatre exercises exploring bodies in space and the relations between them. There was a lunch break, and the afternoon portion of the workshop generally focused on transforming the materials from the first part of the workshop in some way, considering a change to the objects and materials as well as the relations between them.

Radley has argued that visual methods do not make any one voice audible or any one vision visible.[32] Their strength is not in being a better or worse representation of a person's experience but rather in the different *versions* of that experience that are brought to the fore. We were aware in designing the workshops that we could not make every aspect of the experience of chronic pain and the difficulties of communicating it visible. In particular, we did not have time for each person to give an extended narrative around their personal experience of pain, its diagnosis or misdiagnosis, and treatment. Moreover, providing this space at the beginning of the workshop would have served to highlight divisions and distinctions between those with pain and those without. We instead began each workshop by focusing on something related to the workshops themselves, such as participants' experiences with art and creativity, the objects they had brought to represent pain, or what they had been thinking on the way there that morning. As we have argued elsewhere,[33] this had the effect of decentralising the narrative structure of the workshops so that, while individual stories of pain experience were told, they were told relationally, in dialogue with others and in aid of building or producing something together.

One of the workshops' achievements was in moving beyond the common dualism of real/unreal that plagues chronic pain communication.[34,35,36] By using arts materials—images, drawings and sounds, among others—to produce versions of pain, pain came to have a visible or audible reality outside the sufferer. Moreover, this was a reality that was produced by the person with pain, not by a biomedical system intent on diagnosis or treatment. Through this, we were able to move past debates about the causes of pain or the extent to which it was supported or reinforced by structures of an individual's psyche. The workshops generated wider questions about pain, negotiated, debated and contested within the workshop space: Do you see pain as something inside you or as something that comes from outside? Do you find it more helpful to tune into it, building awareness, or to shut it out, abstracting yourself from it? Is the pain an inevitable part of yourself? How and to what extent has pain shaped your personhood? Can there be a 'you' without pain?

Again, there were limits to these methods: producing drawings and using visual art materials, for instance, was more accessible to those with previous artistic training, and not all participants produced aesthetically elegant, engaging or legible images. This is not to negate the value of these images as a particular imagining of pain, but it does make their analytic interpretation more complex, and means they may not lend themselves well to being displayed outside the workshop context. Technologies of digital photography are widely accessible and available, but again, producing good images requires accrued technical skill which goes beyond simply operating a camera phone. The skill of communicating pain through these methods, in ways that are accessible to others, requires facilitation. It is not a *fait accompli*. The mere fact of having pain does not predispose one to produce good art related to pain. Indeed, pain can halt artistic expression as much or more than it enables it.[37]

The methodological choices we made in this project aimed to produce collective versions of pain communication and to see pain as relational, rather than as stuck inside the sufferer, trying more or less successfully to get out. Our focus was therefore on making something with and through pain—using pain as a material—rather than on how difficult pain is to communicate. This is not to deny the many accounts of how pain is, indeed, difficult to communicate, particularly in a clinical context. Nor does it deny the tremendous value of narratives and the importance of people with pain being able to tell their own stories.[38,39] Rather, our work highlighted that no one method of producing versions of pain tells the whole and complete story. Our methods circumscribe at the same time as they document these stories. Alternative methods, producing alternative versions, are important, as is hearing these versions in dialogue with one another.

Ways of Travelling Through Painscapes

Each of the methodological paths through pain that I have outlined above is a particular way of travelling, a version that makes visible or audible particular realities about pain. These paths have focused on the experience of having pain, whether as part of the context of employment that depends in part on one's ability to determine whether everyday pains have gone 'too far' or not, or for those with chronic pain where pain is an overwhelming daily reality. In both cases, pain is a limit, but in the first case there is a degree of control, while in the second, pain takes away control, preventing and limiting daily activities, social interactions and relations.

Obviously, there are significant differences in the experiences of dancers working through pain, who navigate the delicate boundary between 'good' training pain and 'bad' injury pain on a daily basis, and people with chronic pain, whose experience of pain has usually come to them unbidden and unexpectedly. Amongst chronically injured dancers there were stories of unsuccessfully navigating that boundary, where pushing too far and for too long left them suffering persistent, unremitting pain. There were also those who worked in dance despite chronic injury or disability, whose daily experiences of pain and pushing against the limits of their body might be more analogous to those of people with chronic pain. Many dancers, however, had yet to learn the brutal lessons pain teaches those who must suffer it on a regular basis.

Common to all the projects I sketched above is an emphasis on the visual, and on producing things related to pain: a body map, a line drawing, a sculpted figure, a digital image, a soundscape. Producing something outside the self, something that could be referred to in discussions and used as a common reference point, gave pain a materiality it otherwise lacked. Yet it materialised pain in particular ways, making particular things visible: none of these methods captures everything there is to say about pain communication. Rather, they enable and enact certain forms of pain communication.

A growing body of work in science and technology studies (STS) has documented the role of method in co-constituting its findings, both in science and medicine[40,41,42] and in social science.[43,44,45] John Law makes the argument that 'Method, as we usually imagine it, is a system for offering more or less bankable guarantees. It hopes to guide us more or less quickly and securely to our destination, a destination that is taken to be knowledge about the processes at work in a single world'.[46] He argues that method has been reluctant to embrace multiplicity and uncertainty, suggesting that '(social) science should also be trying to make and know realities that are vague and indefinite *because much of the world is enacted in that way*'.[47] For Law, this is best performed through thinking of methods as assemblages rather than linear paths. A method assemblage includes not only what is present or made visible but also what is absent and what is othered 'because, while necessary to presence, it is not or cannot be made manifest'.[48] To go back to the metaphor of method as a way of travelling, a method assemblage would thus consider not only the choices made along the route taken but also the routes not taken, and the routes which were, for one reason or another, inaccessible, out of reach. This is about more than simply considering the limitations of one's research: it is about embracing ambiguity. Law and Urry refer to method in this context as performative: it produces a particular reality at the same time as documenting it.[44] If our methods perform particular realities, we can also make choices—what Barad terms 'agential cuts'—about the realities we produce.[41] Lury and Wakeford's notion of 'inventive methods' provides a similar mode of travel, embracing uncertainty, seeing methods as devices which do things, whose 'use is always oriented towards making a difference'.[49]

Recognising that method produces as well as documents realities is not in any way to deny the reality of pain or the versions of pain produced by methods, whether in the form of standardised pain tools or the more open-ended qualitative and visual methods I have described above. There are good reasons for seeking standardised tools with which to measure pain. As Melzack points out, the McGill Pain Questionnaire is indeed a major advancement on pain scales which define pain only as a number, without recognising the variation in sensation.[10] Recognising that method is performative means accepting the complexity of pain, and that no version is complete on its own. It also means making a commitment to making a difference, to recognising the way that methods carve out and delimit particular versions of pain, and considering what might be left out, absent or othered in these versions. This is challenging, inasmuch as it means embracing a less stable, reproducible version of method and the realities it describes.

The chapters in this volume have focused on a range of methodological pathways, whether via online communication and dissemination of information (Newhouse, Atherton and Ziebland); through visual images in digital contexts (Pardo; Morcate) or clinical ones (Padfield & Zakrzewska; O'Shea, Wilkinson and Jones); through poetry (Rosen) or prose (Bending); through theatrical performance (Goldingay) or the logics of autoimmunity (Andrews). Together, they map disparate paths through painscapes, intersecting at some points, diverging at others. They map territories less often described in medical accounts of pain: territories of everyday connections and empathies alongside and often in contrast to the politics of medical knowledge and power in clinical encounters. They provide alternative modes of attunement, communicative frameworks that work outside of, but also parallel to, the rating scales and predefined terms that so often characterise pain. Together they serve to illustrate pain's diversity and multiplicity, and to suggest multiple ways of travelling through the painscape.

Acknowledgements *Pain and Injury in a Cultural Context: Dancers' Embodied Understandings and Visual Mapping* was funded by the Arts and Humanities Research Council from 2005–2007. *Pain and Visual Mapping* was supported by Trinity College Dublin's Arts Humanities and Social Sciences Benefactions Fund in 2009. *Communicating Chronic Pain: Interdisicplinary Strategies for Non-Textual Data* was funded by the Economic and Social Research Council via the National Centre for Research Methods, 2013–2014. I am grateful to these funders for their support. I also acknowledge the contributions of my collaborators and co-investigators on these projects, in particular Helen Thomas, PI of *Pain and Injury in a Cultural Context*. The CCP workshops would not have been possible without the workshop leaders: Duncan Hodkinson and Rachael Allen, Deborah Padfield and Yoshi Inada, Richard Crow and Steven Lyons, and Nelly Alfandari and Mara Ferreri. Many thanks also to the participants who shared their stories, drawings, insights and artwork across these three projects.

Notes

1. Appadurai, Arjun. "Disjuncture and Difference in the Global Cultural Economy." *Theory, Culture & Society* 7, no. 2 (1990): 295–310, 296.
2. Scarry, Elaine. *The Body in Pain: The Making and Unmaking of the World* (USA: Oxford University Press, 1985), 4.
3. Ibid.
4. Bending, Lucy. *The Representation of Bodily Pain in Late Nineteenth-Century English Culture* (Oxford: Clarendon Press, 2000).
5. Bourke, Joanna. *The Story of Pain: From Prayer to Painkillers* (New York, NY: Oxford University Press, 2014).
6. Crawford, Cassandra S. "From Pleasure to Pain: The Role of the MPQ in the Language of Phantom Limb Pain." *Social Science & Medicine* 69, no. 5 (2009): 655–661.
7. Bourke, Joanna. *The Story of Pain: From Prayer to Painkillers* (New York, NY: Oxford University Press, 2014), 6.
8. Ibid., 68.
9. Melzack, Ronald, and P. D. Wall. "The Challenge of Pain (Rev. ed.)." In *Markham, ON: Penguin Books* (1988), 37.
10. Melzack, Ronald. "The McGill Pain Questionnaire: Major Properties and Scoring Methods." *Pain* 1, no. 3 (1975): 277–299.
11. Melzack, Ronald. "The Short-Form McGill Pain Questionnaire." *Pain* 30, no. 2 (1987): 191–197.

12. Melzack, Ronald, and P. D. Wall. "The Challenge of Pain (Rev. ed.)." *Markham, ON: Penguin Books* (1988), 37.
13. Bieri, Daiva, Robert A. Reeve, G. David Champion, Louise Addicoat, and John B. Ziegler. "The Faces Pain Scale for the Self-assessment of the Severity of Pain Experienced by Children: Development, Initial Validation, and Preliminary Investigation for Ratio Scale Properties." *Pain* 41, no. 2 (1990): 139–150.
14. Crawford, Cassandra S. "From Pleasure to Pain: The Role of the MPQ in the Language of Phantom Limb Pain." *Social Science & Medicine* 69, no. 5 (2009): 655–661, 661.
15. Crawford, Cassandra S. "From Pleasure to Pain: The Role of the MPQ in the Language of Phantom Limb Pain." *Social Science & Medicine* 69, no. 5 (2009): 655–661, 658.
16. De Souza, Lorraine H., and Andrew O. Frank. "Subjective Pain Experience of People with Chronic Back Pain." *Physiotherapy Research International* 5, no. 4 (2000): 207–219.
17. Williams, Amanda C. de C., Huw Talfryn Oakley Davies, and Yasmin Chadury. "Simple Pain Rating Scales Hide Complex Idiosyncratic Meanings." *Pain* 85, no. 3 (2000): 457–463.
18. Smith, Marion V. "Pain Experience and the Imagined Researcher." *Sociology of Health & Illness* 30, no. 7 (2008): 992–1006.
19. Litcher-Kelly, Leighann, Sharon A. Martino, Joan E. Broderick, and Arthur A. Stone. "A Systematic Review of Measures Used to Assess Chronic Musculoskeletal Pain in Clinical and Randomized Controlled Clinical Trials." *The Journal of Pain* 8, no. 12 (2007): 906–991.
20. Heshusius, Lous. *Inside Chronic Pain: An Intimate and Critical Account* (Cornell University Press, 2013), 7.
21. Price, Donald D., Patricia A. McGrath, Amir Rafii, and Barbara Buckingham. "The Validation of Visual Analogue Scales as Ratio Scale Measures for Chronic and Experimental Pain." *Pain* 17, no. 1 (1983): 45–56.
22. Schott, Geoffrey D. "The Cartography of Pain: The Evolving Contribution of Pain Maps." *European Journal of Pain* (2010).
23. Law, John. *After Method: Mess in Social Science Research* (Routledge, 2004).
24. Laws, Helen, and Joanna Apps. *Fit to Dance 2: Report of the Second National Inquiry into Dancers' Health and Injury in the UK* (Dance UK, 2005).

25. Brinson, Peter, and Fiona Dick. *Fit to Dance?: The Report of the National Inquiry into Dancers' Health and Injury* (Calouste Gulbenkian Foundation, 1996).
26. Solomon, R., and L. Micheli. "Concepts in the Prevention of Dance Injuries: A Survey and Analysis." In *The Dancer as Athlete: The 1984 Olympic Scientific Congress Proceedings*, vol. 8, pp. 201–212, 1986.
27. All names are pseudonyms.
28. Gabbe, Belinda J., Caroline F. Finch, Kim L. Bennell, and H. Wajswelner. "How Valid is a Self Reported 12 Month Sports Injury History?" *British Journal of Sports Medicine* 37, no. 6 (2003): 545–547.
29. Tarr, Jen, and Helen Thomas. "Mapping Embodiment: Methodologies for Representing Pain and Injury." *Qualitative Research* 11, no. 2 (2011): 141–157.
30. Gonzalez-Polledo, Elena. "Chronic Media Worlds: Social Media and the Problem of Pain Communication on Tumblr." *Social Media + Society* 2, no. 1 (2016): 2056305116628887.
31. Gonzalez-Polledo, Elena, and Jen Tarr. "The Thing About Pain: The Remaking of Illness Narratives in Chronic Pain Expressions on Social Media." *New Media & Society* 18, no. 8 (2016): 1455–1472.
32. Radley, Alan. "What People Do with Pictures." *Visual Studies* 25, no. 3 (2010): 268–279.
33. Tarr, Jen, Elena Gonzalez-Polledo, and Flora Cornish. "On Liveness: Using Arts Workshops as a Research Method." *Qualitative Research* (2017). doi:10.1177/1468794117694219.
34. Bendelow, Gillian A., and Simon J. Williams. "Transcending the Dualisms: Towards a Sociology of Pain." *Sociology of Health & Illness* 17, no. 2 (1995): 139–165.
35. Kenny, Dianna T. "Constructions of Chronic Pain in Doctor–Patient Relationships: Bridging the Communication Chasm." *Patient Education and Counseling* 52, no. 3 (2004): 297–305.
36. Kugelmann, Robert. "Complaining About Chronic Pain." *Social Science & Medicine* 49, no. 12 (1999): 1663–1676.
37. Vick, Randy M., and Kathy Sexton-Radek. "Art and Migraine: Researching the Relationship Between Artmaking and Pain Experience." *Art Therapy* 22, no. 4 (2005): 193–204.
38. Charon R. *Narrative Medicine: Honoring the Stories of Illness* (New York; Oxford: Oxford University Press, 2006).
39. Frank, Arthur W. *The Wounded Storyteller: Body, Illness and Ethics* (Chicago; London: University of Chicago Press, 1995).

40. Haraway, Donna Jeanne. *Modest—Witness@ Second—Millennium. FemaleMan—Meets—OncoMouse: Feminism and Technoscience* (Psychology Press, 1997).
41. Barad, Karen. *Meeting the Universe Halfway: Quantum Physics and the Entanglement of Matter and Meaning* (Duke University Press, 2007).
42. Mol, Annemarie. *The Body Multiple: Ontology in Medical Practice* (Duke University Press, 2002).
43. Law, John. *After Method: Mess in Social Science Research* (Routledge, 2004).
44. Law, John, and John Urry. "Enacting the Social." *Economy and Society* 33, no. 3 (2004): 390–410.
45. Lury, Celia, and Nina Wakeford, eds. *Inventive Methods: The Happening of the Social* (Routledge, 2012).
46. Law, 9.
47. Ibid., 14.
48. Ibid., 84.
49. Lury, Celia, and Nina Wakeford, eds. *Inventive Methods: The Happening of the Social* (Routledge, 2012), 11.

Jen Tarr is Assistant Professor of Research Methodology in the Department of Methodology at the LSE. She is a health sociologist whose research and teaching focus on qualitative methods, particularly visual and other sensory approaches. Her research interests include the sociology of pain, movement practices such as dance and the use of somatics, and complementary and alternative medicine techniques. She has published in journals such as *Qualitative Research* and *Sociology of Health & Illness*.

Index[1]

A

Acute illness, 65
Acute pain, 2, 88, 89
Aesthetics, 5, 10, 15, 48, 116, 144, 222, 225n33
Affect, 7, 20n37, 78, 84, 98, 107, 142, 158, 161, 184, 186–188, 233
Ahmed, Sarah, 98, 99, 105n48, 105n50
Alzheimer's, 159, 161–164, 166, 170–172
American Civil War, 12, 25
Anaesthesia, 1, 2, 32
Anaesthetics, 2
Appadurai, Arjun, 11, 229, 245n1
Archives, 91, 130
Arthritis, 9, 16, 85, 93, 184–190, 194, 197, 238

Articulation (pain), 26, 86
Attention, 9–11, 26, 28, 32–34, 62, 63, 84, 102, 158, 171
Attunement, 12, 244
Authenticity, 13, 61–78, 137
Autobiography, 5, 14, 55, 58, 86, 158, 163
Autoimmunity, 13, 14, 85–90, 95, 99–101, 102n7, 103n12, 244
Autopoiesis, 89–94, 100, 104n26

B

Barad, Karen, 244, 248n41
Becoming, 28, 47, 85, 90, 98, 122, 139, 141, 184, 213, 233
Bendelow, Gillian, 3, 19n19, 19n20, 247n34

[1]Note: Page numbers followed by "n" refers to notes.

Berlant, Lauren, 6, 7, 20n37, 20n38, 20n39, 95, 96, 98, 99, 101, 104n36, 105n38, 105n39, 105n49, 105n51
Binaries
  acute versus chronic, 65
  Cartesian, 206
Biro, David, 10, 18n14, 22n57, 205, 206, 223n6, 223n14, 224n15
Boal, Augusto, 73, 74, 80n27
Body scanning, 236
Bourke, Joanna, 1, 2, 17n2, 17n6, 28, 39, 205, 206, 223n7, 224n16, 230, 231, 245n5, 245n7
Brief Pain Inventory, 209
Bury, Michael, 143, 151n5

C

Care, 3, 6, 27, 33, 36, 63, 65, 66, 76, 86, 88, 89, 93, 97, 98, 112, 133, 138–143, 147, 149, 150, 170, 185, 187, 207
Carel, Havi, 9, 10, 21n49, 22n53, 22n54, 22n55
Casualty (BBC drama), 64, 65
Charon, Rita, 20n28, 21n44, 205, 207, 223n5, 247n38
Chronic pain, 2–4, 7, 8, 13, 15, 16, 17n10, 18n12, 19n22, 42–46, 48–50, 55, 57–59, 60n7, 61, 89, 94–100, 130–132, 134–137, 140, 141, 143–150, 190, 191, 208–212, 220, 222, 229, 233, 242–245

Chronic pain, v, 235
Church, 53, 67
Clinical photography, 15
Clinical relations, 9, 12
Communicating Chronic Pain, v, vi, 59, 60n7, 240
Crawford, Cassandra, 231, 245n6, 246n14, 246n15
Cripistemology, 97, 100
Crohn's disease, 12, 42
Cromwell, Oliver, 53, 60n13
Culture, 3, 8, 13, 14, 18n14, 42, 43, 45, 51–54, 56–58, 61, 63–66, 68, 69, 71, 98, 164, 167, 169, 184, 230

D

Dance, 68, 236, 243
Daniels, Maja, 170
Das, Veena, 11, 20n36, 22n63, 22n64
Death, 1, 14, 97, 165, 166
  death images, 107
Debility, 96, 97
Deconstruction, 84, 88, 93, 94, 101, 103n15
Dementia, 161, 162, 164, 170, 171
Depardon, Raymond, 162, 169, 176n19, 181n69, 181n70
Derrida, Jacques, 13, 87, 88, 90–93, 101, 102n1, 102n2, 102n5, 102n6, 102n7, 103n9, 103n10, 103n12, 103n18, 103n22, 104n23, 104n24, 104n30, 104n32, 104n33, 105n53
Dickinson, Emily, 44

Différance, 88, 90
Disability, 4, 6, 8, 9, 20n35, 21n47, 21n48, 86, 94, 96, 97, 174, 190, 225n41, 237, 238, 240, 243
Doctor–patient relationship
  interaction, 61, 64, 68, 74
  roles, 61, 70

E

Empathy, 42–46, 53, 54, 56–58, 72, 74–77, 217, 244
Empowerment, 73, 135, 147
Epistemic justice, 22n55
Ethics, 8–11, 20n27, 21n44, 54, 160, 162
Exhibiting pain, 107–123
Experience, 1, 26, 42, 62, 84, 108, 129, 159, 183, 206, 231
  of pain, 25, 42, 61, 83, 107, 130

F

Face2face, 207, 212–215, 218, 219, 221–224
Fibromyalgia, 8, 9, 19n22, 131, 132, 141
Forum Theatre, 73–75
Freire, Paulo, 74, 80n27

H

Health services, 130, 131, 138–142, 164, 180n64
Heshusius, Lous, 233, 246n20
Homo economicus, 94, 95

Huertas, Rafael, 167, 168, 178n33, 178n34, 180n61, 180n65
Humoral physiology, 53
Hypochondria, 69

I

Iconography, 157, 159, 160, 167, 168, 173
Identity, 9, 13, 16, 20n38, 48, 52, 98, 121, 132, 134, 136, 137, 172, 184, 221–223
Illness, 34, 42, 62, 85, 108, 129, 207
Illness narratives, 5, 6, 8, 9, 144, 158, 160, 163
Imagination, 11, 17, 40, 49–51, 57, 69, 198
Immune system, 85, 87, 89–92, 102n7, 103n20
Inclusion, 87, 98
Injury, 3, 25, 28, 29, 33, 43, 50, 93, 134, 188, 206, 231, 236–240, 242, 243
Instagram, 122, 145, 159, 160, 171
Intentionality, 13, 49–51
Interfaces, 11, 13, 15, 18n16, 141
Internet, 117
  cyberchondria, 141
  digital resources, 130, 131, 148, 149
  online communication, 136, 244
  platforms, 119, 122, 138
  memorial platform, 117
Ishiuchi, Miyako, 114, 115, 118
Isolation, 43, 48, 55, 57, 88, 135, 137, 144, 162, 164, 172, 209, 210, 214

J

Jackson, Jean, 7, 8, 21n40, 21n41, 21n42
Jain, Lochlann, 6, 20n34
Journalism, 161
Jurecic, Ann, 5, 6, 20n29, 20n30

K

Keats, John, 51
Keen, William, 27, 28
Kirchuk, Alejandro, 170
Kleinman, Arthur, 4, 18n17, 19n24, 21n40, 21n46, 22n63, 80n23, 177n27, 207, 226n19

L

Language, v, 5, 10, 12, 15, 16, 25–46, 49–55, 57–59, 68, 85, 89, 96, 104n27, 157, 162, 165, 189, 198, 200, 203, 205, 206, 210–217, 222, 231–236
Law, John, 243, 246n23, 248n43, 248n44
Listening, 10, 12, 14, 16, 18n14, 26, 38
Luhmann, Niklas, 92, 93, 95, 104n25, 104n26, 104n30, 104n35

M

Malingering, 34, 150
Manderson, Lenore, 4, 18n13, 19n21, 20n35
Materiality, 9, 71, 217, 243
Maturana, Humberto, 89, 92, 103n16, 104n28

Matzinger, Polly, 91, 103n21
McGill Pain Questionnaire (MPQ), 10, 206, 209, 232, 239, 244
 in translation, 231
Mental illness, 15, 157
Merendino, Angelo, 118–122
Messiness, 234
Metaphor, 3, 43, 50, 53–58, 84, 87, 93, 104n27, 208, 209, 212, 213, 230, 243
Mitchell, Silas Weir, 12, 25
Molière, 68–70
Moore, Pete, 62, 79n9
Morehouse, George, 27, 28, 34
Morris, David, 223n5, 226n50, 226n51
Moscoso, Javier, 17n8, 164, 168, 180n63
Multiplicity, 102, 219, 234, 243, 244

N

Narratives
 and history, 12
 normative narratives, 87, 98
Negative capability, 51
NHS, 186, 222
Numerical Rating Scale, 209, 231, 233
Nutbeam, Don, 142, 152n24

O

O'Halloran, Kenneth, 170
Organism, 85, 89–92, 104n26, 195
 body-as-organism, 89
Osteoarthritis, 63, 131, 140, 143, 184, 185, 188, 189, 194, 197, 201, 238, 239

P

Pain environments, 7, 13, 14, 89, 95, 184, 213, 231
Pain facts, 2, 38, 116, 123, 131, 132, 215, 232, 241
  pain research, 233
Pain images, 15–16
  pain drawings, 233, 239
Pain journey, 220
Pain scale, 10, 232, 244
Painscapes, vi, 1–17
Parsons, Talcott, 61, 71
Participation, 148, 183, 185
Patients
  doctor–patient dynamics, 130
  patient expertise, 77
  prosumers, 15, 148
Patsavas, Alyson, 97, 98, 100, 105n41, 105n43
Perceptions of Pain, 212–214, 219
Performance, 13, 26, 28, 31, 61, 66–76, 198, 208, 231, 244
  performance studies, 64, 66, 71
Performativity, 53, 73, 243, 244
Perkins-Gilman, Charlotte, 27
Pernick, Martin, 1, 17n3, 17n4
Personae, 61
Pharmakon, 88, 90
Phenomenology, 22n54, 234
Philosophy, 4, 11, 13, 71
Phonography, 171
Photo art projects, 108
Photo-elicitation, 206
Photography, v, vi, 14–16, 45, 107, 110, 123, 157–184, 195, 197, 199, 215, 221, 240, 241
  grieving image, 109
Photojournalism, 15, 158, 159, 168–171
Physiology, 1, 53, 230

Placebo, 64, 72
Poetry, 5, 12, 42, 44–46, 48, 49, 51–55, 244
Politics, 4, 6, 9, 36, 39, 52, 95, 100, 101, 244
  political intervention, 15
Polysemy, 219
Postbiomedical, 9
Postcolonial, 72
Posthuman, 94
Post-phenomenology, 4, 16
Puar, Jasbir, 96, 97, 105n40, 105n42

R

Radley, Alan, 207, 215, 225n32, 225n33, 226n28, 226n29, 226n30, 226n60, 226n61, 227n64, 240, 247n32
Readability, 98, 132
Recognition, 3, 9, 13, 28, 35, 59, 135, 234
Representation, 5, 10, 13–16, 35, 42, 49, 56, 71, 98, 109–111, 117, 158–162, 165, 167–169, 171, 173, 208, 220, 233, 240
Resistance, 5, 13, 42, 44, 45, 48, 57, 83, 100, 145, 162, 230, 233

S

Science & technology studies (STS), 243
Self
  self-care, 63, 84
  selfhood, 6
  self in pain, 84
  self-referentiality, 92, 163
  subject of pain, 39, 46

Sick role, 61, 71
Skeptics, 53
Smith-Morris, Carolyn, 4, 19n21, 20n35
Sontag, Susan, 43, 45, 56, 57, 59n1, 60n5, 124n4, 162, 165, 166, 169, 172, 176n17, 179n50, 180n44, 180n45, 180n46, 180n47, 227n69
Spence, Jo, 207, 216, 226n26, 226n27, 226n28
Spinoza, Baruch, 54
Stahl, Devan, 221, 227n73, 227n74
Stigmatization, 157–159, 173
Story, vi, 5, 8, 9, 12, 21n52, 31, 35, 36, 39, 63–66, 70, 77, 99, 100, 107, 110, 113, 115–123, 130–132, 141–146, 172, 207, 214, 241, 242
Suffering, 1, 2, 4, 14, 25, 42, 43, 47, 58, 59, 70, 84, 86–89, 91, 94–101, 107, 108, 110, 114, 141, 164, 171, 173, 185, 186, 222, 243
Support
 support networks, 134
 support relationships, 130
Surgery, 29, 65, 116, 133, 139, 187, 188, 216, 219, 236
Systems theory, 84, 89, 92–96, 101, 104n27

T
Temporality
 futurity, 14
 present, 12

Teubner, Gunter, 93, 104n30
Toledano, Philip, 117, 118, 126n21, 126n22, 126n23, 172, 181n81, 181n82
Torture, 36, 43, 50, 88
Translation, 26, 39, 68, 98
Trauma, 6, 26, 43, 64, 65, 85, 97, 99, 101, 134, 207

V
Varela, Francisco, 89, 92, 103n16, 103n20, 104n28
Verbal Rating Scale, 209
Violence, 43, 48, 57, 58, 91–94, 96, 99, 100, 102, 160, 161, 174
Visibility, 14, 15, 27, 108, 159, 171
Visual Analogue Scale, 209, 231–233
Vocabulary, 10, 140, 142, 143, 161, 211, 213
Vogl, Joseph, 94, 95, 104n34
Voice, 15, 27, 32, 37, 46, 49, 59, 120, 122, 133, 171, 240

W
Welfare, 43, 45
Witnessing, 11, 210, 211
Wyke, Sally, 131, 134, 138, 145, 150n1, 151n3

Z
Ziebland, Sue, v, 15, 131, 134, 138, 145, 150n1, 151n3, 244

The manufacturer's authorised representative in the EU is Springer Nature Customer Service Centre GmbH, Europaplatz 3, 69115 Heidelberg, Germany. If you have any concerns regarding our products, please contact ProductSafety@springernature.com

Printed and bound by CPI Group (UK) Ltd, Croydon, CR0 4YY

23/03/2026

02076663-0004